SomatoEmotional Release®

Other books by Dr. Upledger include:

CranioSacral Therapy

CranioSacral Therapy II: Beyond the Dura

SomatoEmotional Release and Beyond

A Brain Is Born: Exploring the Birth and Development of the Central Nervous System

Your Inner Physician and You

CranioSacral Therapy: Touchstone for Natural Healing

SomatoEmotional Release®

Deciphering the Language of Life

John E. Upledger, D.O., O.M.M.

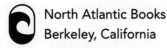 North Atlantic Books
Berkeley, California

UI Enterprises
Palm Beach Gardens, Florida

Published by

North Atlantic Books
P.O. Box 12327
Berkeley, California 94712

UI Enterprises
11211 Prosperity Farms Road, Ste. D-325
Palm Beach Gardens, Florida 33410

Cover and book design by Paula Morrison

Printed in the United States of America

SomatoEmotional Release: Deciphering the Language of Life is sponsored by the Society for the Study of Native Arts and Sciences, a nonprofit educational corporation whose goals are to develop an educational and cross-cultural perspective linking various scientific, social, and artistic fields; to nurture a holistic view of arts, sciences, humanities, and healing; and to publish and distribute literature on the relationship of mind, body, and nature.

North Atlantic Books' publications are available through most bookstores. For further information, call 800-337-2665 or visit our website at www.northatlanticbooks.com.

Substantial discounts on bulk quantities are available to corporations, professional associations, and other organizations. For details and discount information, contact our special sales department.

Library of Congress Cataloging-in-Publication Data
Upledger, John E., 1932-
    SomatoEmotional release : deciphering the language of life / by John
E. Upledger ; foreword by Richard Grossinger.
        p. ; cm.
    Includes index.
    ISBN 1-55643-412-X (pbk.)
    1. Craniosacral therapy.
    [DNLM: 1. Manipulation, Orthopedic—methods. 2. Psychophysiologic
Disorders—therapy. 3. Emotions. 4. Osteopathic Medicine—methods. WM
90 U67s 2002] I. Title.
    RZ399.C73 U67 2002

                                                                2002008149

1 2 3 4 5 6 7 8 9 / 07 06 05 04 03 02

Important Note

Medical knowledge is ever changing. As new research and clinical experience broaden our knowledge, changes in treatment and drug therapy may be required. The authors and editors of the material herein have consulted sources believed to be reliable in their efforts to provide information that is complete and in accordance with the standards accepted at the time of publication.

However, the authors, editors, publisher, or any other parties who have been involved in the preparation of this work, do not warrant the information contained herein and are not responsible for any errors or omissions resulting from use of such information.

Readers are encouraged to confirm the information contained herein with other sources to best suit their particular situations.

Some of the product names, patents, and registered designs referred to in this book are in fact registered trademarks or proprietary names, even though specific reference to this fact is not always made in the text. Therefore, the appearance of a name without designation as proprietary is not to be construed as a representation by the publisher that it is in the public domain.

Contents

Foreword

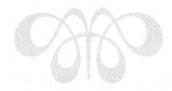

When John Upledger asked me to write the introduction to this book, I thought, "I'm the wrong person. First of all, I'm the publisher; I'm not the traditional outside expert to lend credibility. We need someone with more name recognition, ideally in the medical field. Plus, John has already written an introduction to one of my books, so we might be accused of being in cahoots." These points aside, however, I consider it an honor and a gift to be able to introduce this book.

John Upledger is the real thing. He is a healer in an age of not only epidemic disease but epidemic quackery—sadly, a quackery that is lodged as trenchantly in the core of the medical establishment as in any alternative arena. He is also a sober and honest man among inflaters and self-promoters, a seer among sophists. By that I mean that he makes no purely intellectual or theoretical claim to explanations or sole authority; he observes and follows the signs and clues of an elusive natural world and the organisms that inhabit it. Contrary to popular opinion, empiricism is a territory that physics and biochemistry have far from locked up.

There are plenty of physicians, of both conventional allopathic bent and a range of unorthodox persuasions, who tell us how things are—how creatures congeal from raw material (or spirit) and then function; how diseases arise, how they should be identified and treated. Those in the allopathic camp point to concrete pathogen vectors, discrete tissue sites; their treatments are usually surgical procedures and drugs. Those in the alternative and complementary camps cite a medley of energies and transpersonal forces; they treat by affirmations, microdoses, breath, archetypes, and manual techniques. John

Upledger is in neither camp; he remains absolutely empirical, open and receptive to any technique or paradigm that succeeds, regardless of its origin or pedigree, yet suffering no fools. That is, though he assays energy fields and elemental forces in the manner of traditional Chinese medicine or Ayurveda, he is equally respectful of cell life, tissue pathologies, autopsies, and skillful surgical intervention. He does not accede uncritically to inflations of New Age healers and spiritualists any more than he adheres to orthodox medical categories. Thus, he is in the unusual position of being a trained scientist and doctor who regards all entities and agencies—cosmic, psychic, or visceral—that operate within the human domain and affect the health of individuals, singly and collectively.

Upledger is in fact an extremely well-trained physician. In an Olympics of anatomy, surgery, neuropsychiatry, and pharmacy, he would probably give most present-day medical-school graduates and research physicians a run for their money. He is also more outcome-oriented than most HMO doctors who are balancing legal and economic imperatives and religiously staying within the bounds of sanctioned disease categories and remedies. His strength lies in results more than theory—despite the fact that he is one of the great theoreticians of our time. When he proposes holistic and energetic cures, he does so from the standpoint of one who has carried out extensive dissections and surgeries and has diagnosed and treated the full array of baffling and life-threatening conditions, while attending the young, the old, and all the stages of men and women in between during a decades-long stint in family medicine. This distinguished medical career pre-dated much of his exploration of the innovative methods portrayed in this book.

At the same time, Upledger seeks no appointment as either the king's physician or the leader of a separatist medical insurgency. It is notable in this regard that he chose to resign a consultancy at The National Institutes of Health (Office of Alternative Medicine) because he did not want to waste time helping to devise clinical trials for methods that, to his satisfaction, worked fine. He realized that statistical or causal proof for some key modalities might be near impossible to attain in the short run, and he could not afford the luxury of trying to devise the appropriate protocols when so many sick people needed to be helped. Instead, he put his time into bringing innovative healing techniques to some of the more neglected victims of society—victims of torture, veterans with post-traumatic stress disorder, newborns in hospitals, children with Down's syndrome and autism, and youth in school systems. Working with dolphins, he also pioneered protocols of trans-species healing and thus tried to overcome the barrier of anthropomorphism that otherwise condemns the human species to being alone on this planet.

Mainstream medical science these days emphasizes programs of diagnosis and treatment that conceptually dismember the human organism (and life itself) into smaller and smaller machinelike, thermochemical bits. A clinician or researcher is presumed to be most modern and closest to first causes when he or she is operating on a molecular level. Diseases are often considered untreatable or incurable for reasons of genetic determinism or molecular fatalism. Furthermore, even when potentially fruitful, allopathic treatment is limited to literal attacks upon pathology. Human beings become mere repositories of random, dissociative, exogenous ailments. There is no link between our sentience and our biological functioning. As essentially inert and nonsentient motes, neither molecules nor the cells they comprise (which conduct their metabolism) can be altered other than by concrete interference in and deterrence of their patterns. These patterns are considered entropic and inevitable unless deterred and mechanically reprogrammed.

Such medicine is meant for life forms that totally lack mind and spirit, and lack homeostatic energy processes and synergistic reintegration too. In an era in which advanced technology alone is considered progress, an integral and componential infrastructure rules the medical profession, and any treatment that is holistic is considered suspect and soft because it does not get down to a microscopic and subcellular level, does not reduce the organism to its raw atomistic parts. When cures arise from holistic treatments (whether herbs, palpations, emotional gestalts, or modes of vital energy), they are ascribed to misinterpretation or placebo effect. This entails (as well, by the way) a total misunderstanding of "placebo" and its crucial role in *all* cures.

Speaking recently of media mogul Ted Turner, Bob Wright, C.E.O. of NBC, could have been describing John Upledger with these words: "He sees the obvious before most people do. We all look at the same picture but [he] sees what you don't see. And after he sees it, it becomes obvious to everyone."

What John Upledger sees is a world in which myriad physical, emotional, cognitive, and transpersonal factors converge to create the human sphere. These factors are rarely considered in terms of one another, at least not in a serious medical context. They include— and I want to be careful here not to simplify Dr. Upledger's position or make him seem credulous—paraphysical energies, subliminal and nonconscious codes, and disembodied intelligences. At no point, however, does Upledger make telekinetic or hyperdimensional claims per se; he accepts the spoken (and unspoken) transmissions of the human organism in their own terms—in precisely the terms they present themselves—and follows their intrinsic wisdom. He presumes that an organism's actual signs and voices are more completely organized and deeply imbedded in the ancient network we call life than any imposed external interpretations based on mechanical and purely thermodynamic views of life.

Dr. Upledger does something so obvious and simple that it could be overlooked and yet so radical that it lies outside of any contemporary paradigm—he listens to cells and tissues and tries to respond appropriately. His listening is informed medically, psychospiritually, and probably shamanically too (in the best sense). He is willing to set aside his skepticism and any preexisting belief system and respond to what is happening with the person he is helping. He does not engage in undue speculation or mythodrama. Dr. Upledger is very "nuts and bolts." The organism tells him what's going on, and he responds as best he can. Trying out the obvious and the explicit and following it nonprejudicially to its natural conclusion is, sadly, rare in the world of either medicine or science.

From the standpoint of modality selection, cure, and ultimate personal freedom, it is mainly important to make people well and to give their organisms flexibility and the power to adjust to stress and other assaults on their integrity. We can't solve the riddles of the universe or know exactly whether a "voice" is an entity, an archetype, a Freudian symbol, a metaphor, or even a delusion. As Upledger snapped at me once when I questioned the authenticity of a ploy during a session, "F—— that! Humor me, will you?"

If addressed in the terms in which it arises, a symptom or utterance is engaged authentically and in a venue that best serves both patient and doctor. It is not essential to decide here and now whether we are "born again," "born again and again," or sociobiological automatons living single, arbitrary lives ("Oh, Son of Man, thou canst not know. . . ."). It *is* essential to give the organism the respect it requires in order for it to be willing to get itself well, which means (first and foremost) listening without interrupting.

John Upledger operates from a primary axiom: "Do not yourself become part of the problem you are trying to solve." Most physicians do not even consider this issue because they do not regard the larger fields of intelligences holding together metabolic homeostases in life forms and societies. They make subtle, impeccable feints on surgical and pharmaceutical (material) planes, while they simultaneously blunder through underlying nexuses of resistance nodes (energy cysts) and innate curative motifs (inner physicians) in the body-mind. The tissues may be altered "correctly" in an academic sense and according to the "manufacturer's instructions" for some piece of equipment, but the life context is disturbed; thus, the treatment does not settle and augment itself; it does not permeate the hidden intelligence of the organism in a way that leads to a lasting, spreading, and self-transforming cure.

Upledger's treatments at least speak the language of the organism and initiate a profound and lasting dialogue.

The goal of medicine should be to creatively disorganize an overly rigid or false organismic structure/belief so that the body, mind, and spirit of the life form can reorganize itself creatively in a better, more synergistic fashion. The block to healing lies in an immobilized, often inscrutable bond between resistance and metabolism that requires fresh energy and transduction. The language of cells communicating with one another is intrinsic to the healthy functioning of tissues and organisms; yet that communication system is not necessarily penetrable by pharmaceutical intervention or bioengineering (such as implanting stem cells in diseased tissue to grow replacement parts). Since all cells originated in multipotentiated, holographically projected forerunners, all cells are potentially stem; all cells can respond therapeutically to the invocations of the *inner physician;* all cells can be reintegrated in the complex signalling networks of the body-mind. A creative dialogue, especially one using touch rather than words (or in conjunction with words), can rearrange the biological code tying organ systems and life force together and thus catalyze the *inner physician.*

To Upledger that means *everything* counts—the intention behind the scalpel as well as the scalpel, the thoughts and hidden agendas of a physician, words spoken in the presence of languageless newborns or patients under supposedly full anesthesia, and the mythologies and belief systems lodged not only in the patient's conscious but unconscious dimensions. These are not superfluities and superstitions; a medicine proposed in their terms approaches the level of the ineffable, subatomic bond between mind and body, matter and energy, form and meaning. In that sense, a modernized shamanism in the guise of SomatoEmotional Release might be millennia ahead of both physical medicine and biotechnology in understanding that symbolized entities rule every level of organism and consciousness; otherwise, sentient, autonomous agents made of cells and organelles could not arise in a biosphere. This is what Upledger sees *now* and everyone will one day see—if a human epidemic of materialism and commoditization of life does not ruin this planet first.

John Upledger stands at the dawn of a new era of medicine and a new era of science. He reads the pulse of collective knowledge well, with a kind of tribal savvy and street smarts rather than scientistic or metaphysical system-making. He sees that eventually the laws of thermodynamics, cellular dialogue, Heisenberg's principle of uncertainty, neo-Darwinian and genetic determinisms, chaos theory, and such matters as superstrings and self-constructing systems of autononomous agents comprising biospheres must come together with psi phenomena (telepathy and telekinetics), karmic and reincarnational philosophy, the Freudian unconscious, dreams, chakras, meridians, discarnate intelligence, and the unique poetry and insights that make each of us human, alive, and unique. This is the only way to create a science of the actual universe in which creatures live and thrive. The alternative would be a sterile techno-domain of robots, stellar explosions, global exploitation, and unimaginable cruelty to present and future life forms. Upledger is optimistic enough and confident enough to believe that the universe is big and wise enough eventually to succeed, and that any one person—every single person—can make the whole difference.

Richard Grossinger

Grossinger has a Ph.D. in anthropology and is the author of numerous books, including *Planet Medicine: Origins; Planet Medicine: Modalities; The Night Sky; Embryogenesis: Species, Gender, and Identity;* and *Embryos, Galaxies, and Sentient Beings: How the Universe Makes Life.* His additional writings on SomatoEmotional Release appear in both volumes of *Planet Medicine, Embryogenesis,* and in his essay on somatic therapies and psychoanalysis in *The Body in Psychotherapy,* edited by Don Hanlon Johnson and Ian J. Grand. All of these are published by North Atlantic Books.

Introduction

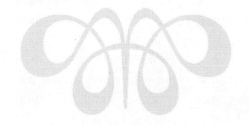

An Overview of CranioSacral Therapy

Most of this book will present specific personal stories and case histories involving the often dramatic ways in which emotion stored in the body can be released to therapeutic effect. Today we know these therapeutic events as SomatoEmotional Release® (SER). SomatoEmotional Release is one of the therapeutic processes we discovered in the late 1970s through our work with CranioSacral Therapy (CST). The latter is actually the "trunk" of a continuously flowering "tree" of therapeutic modalities. We will be writing about many of these modalities as we present SER. But in order to understand any of them, some familiarity with CST is necessary. We will therefore summarize what CST is, its anatomical basis, the rudiments of how it is practiced, and the fundamental principles of its application. We will then be ready to define SER precisely and discuss it in depth.

CranioSacral Therapy is a gentle, minimally invasive method for enhancing the functioning of virtually every system in the body, as well as facilitating the harmonious coordination of body, mind and spirit. These are large claims, but I hope this book will go a long way toward showing why they are justified. In order to see what CST is and why it can influence so many areas of our existence, we first have to understand a bit about the craniosacral system.

The craniosacral system is a coherent physiological system that has only recently come to be recognized as a functioning unit. It is concerned with the production, reabsorption and containment of cerebrospinal fluid. Cerebrospinal fluid is secreted by the brain and provides a fluid environment for the brain and the nervous system. The anatomical parts of the craniosacral system are: the meningeal membranes and the system they form; the bony structures to which the meningeal membranes are attached; other connective tissues intimately related to meningeal membranes; the cerebrospinal fluid itself; and all structures related to it.

The meningeal system envelops the whole brain and spinal cord. It consists of three layers of membrane. The outermost layer is called the "dura mater." It is tough and waterproof. The innermost layer is called the "pia mater." This layer follows every contour and groove of the brain and spinal cord, maintains surface contact with them, and carries many of the blood vessels that service them. The middle layer is the arachnoid membrane. It is a gliding surface between the dura mater and the pia mater. Cerebrospinal fluid flows between each of the layers and serves as a lubricant between them as they move in relation to each other. If these layers stick together in an area, the result is pain. Where the pain is felt depends upon where the membranes are stuck together and whether or not nerves are involved or "pinched" in the stuck areas. Pain can be local or "referred" to a distant point in the body. It is the job of the CranioSacral Therapist to identify areas where membranes are not free to glide and thus are sources of pain and/or dysfunction.

The craniosacral system is intimately related to, influences, and is influenced by the nervous system, the musculoskeletal system, the vascular system, the lymphatic system, the immune system, the endocrine system (the system responsible for the production of hormones), and the respiratory system. The reason that the craniosacral system is so closely related to so many aspects of our physiology has to do with two things: a special pulse or motion characteristic of the craniosacral system, and the communication of this motion to the fascia—the sheets of connective tissue that cover every internal aspect of the human body, its organs and its tissues.

Anterior   Anterior

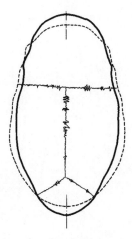   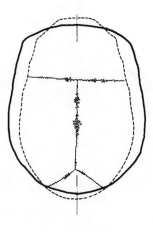

Illustration 0-1A.   Illustration 0-1B.
The skull in extreme extension.   The skull in extreme flexion.

The craniosacral motion is a rhythmic activity that persists through-out life. It occurs in man, other primates, canines, felines, and prob-ably all or most other vertebrates. It is distinct from the motions connected to breathing and cardiovascular activity.

It can be felt externally, most readily on the head or the sacrum. With practice and the development of skill it can be "palpated" (per-ceived through trained touch) anywhere on the body. The cranio-sacral motion is a stable pulse of between six and twelve cycles per minute. It is so stable, in fact, that variations outside of this range are used by the CranioSacral Therapist as indications of pathology.

The rhythmic activity appears at the sacrum as a gentle rocking motion. Its motion can also be felt as a subtle widening and narrow-ing of the head. [See Illustrations 0-1A and B.] The widening phase is called the flexion of the craniosacral system. During flexion, the entire skeletal system rotates in an outward direction. [See Illustration 0-2.] The narrowing is called extension. During the extension phase the head narrows and the whole body rotates inward. [See Illustration 0-3.]

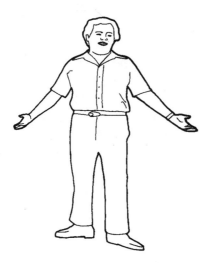

Illustration 0-2.
Whole-body habitus of chronic
craniosacral tension.

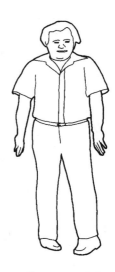

Illustration 0-3.
Whole-body habitus of chronic
craniosacral extension.

There is a neutral zone in each cycle between the end of one phase and the beginning of the next. This can be felt by the practitioner as a slight pause before the physiological forces move into the opposite phase of motion.

The fascia, as I mentioned, is a slightly mobile, laminated sheath of connective tissue that extends continuously throughout the body from head to toe, and covers all of its somatic and visceral structures. By some mechanism, probably via the nervous system, the craniosacral rhythmic motion is normally communicated to the fascia. Since the fascia envelops every organ of the body, the condition of the craniosacral motion can consequently affect and be affected by every organ.

Loss of fascial mobility in any specific area can be used as an aid in the location of the disease process which has caused that lack of mobility.

The CranioSacral Therapist palpates the craniosacral rhythm for rate, amplitude (strength), symmetry (whether, for instance, the rotation during flexion is greater in the right leg than in the left) and quality. Deviations in rate or symmetry indicate pathology. The therapist's training involves learning how to use palpation and the information it makes available under these categories to identify where in the craniosacral system there is a problem. The amount of diagnostic and prognostic information that can be obtained in this way is limited only by the skill and anatomical knowledge of the examiner.

History

CranioSacral Therapy has its origins in osteopathic medicine and the work of William G. Sutherland. While a student of osteopathy in the early 1900s, Sutherland became fascinated by the anatomical design of the bones of the human skull. It seemed to him that they were designed to move, even though he had been taught that skull bones in the normal adult human are fused solidly by calcification and therefore unable to move. Sutherland created an ingenious device that enabled him to study his own cranium and demonstrate to his own satisfaction that the bones of the skull do indeed move. He found that the cranial sutures (the joints between the various bones of the cranium) do fuse—in corpses! Since the crania studied by anatomists were corpse skulls, they naturally believed that cranial bones are immobile. But in the living cranium the sutures are not fused and the bones do move. [See Illustrations 0-4 A and B.]

Once Sutherland became familiar with his own cranial motion he began experimenting on others by gently palpating their heads. Soon he was able to sense a minute rhythmic motion of the cranium. Early on he also found a correlative motion in the sacrum that occurs in synchrony with the motion of the cranium. Sutherland accounted for the synchrony based on the continuity of the dura mater. The dura mater lines the spinal canal and is in the form of a tube. It firmly connects the occiput, which forms part of the base and back of the skull, to the sacrum, with a few bony attachments between. He then developed a model that placed the sphenoid bone as the keystone of the cranium. The sphenoid is the butterfly-shaped bone that forms part of the floor of the skull cavity and part of the sides of the skull just

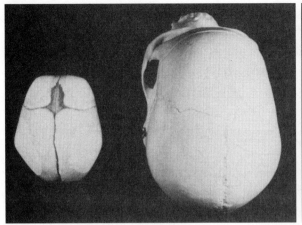

Illustration 0-4A.
Apparent sutural closure in fetal
and adult human skulls.

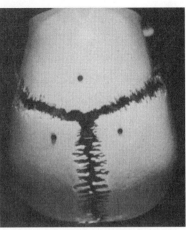

Illustration 0-4B.
"Exploded" human skull
demonstrating non-closure of
sutures.

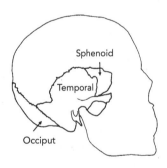

Illustration 0-5.
Relationship among the
sphenoid, temporal and
occiput.

forward of the temple area and back from the corners of the eyes. [See Illustration 0-5.]

Sutherland suggested that the sphenoid moves in response to the circulation of the cerebrospinal fluid and its effect upon the membrane system within the cranium. He thought that the origin of all this motion was the rhythmic contraction and expansion of the system of ventricles in the brain.

Our research has largely supported this model, with the exception of the source of the rhythmic motion. We propose an alternative explanation that we call the "Pressurestat Model." In this model the brain does not actually expand and contract. Rather, it passively responds to hydraulic forces. We hypothesize that the production of cerebrospinal fluid within the ventricular system of the brain is significantly more rapid than its reabsorption back into the venous system within the cranium. There-fore, when fluid production is turned on for a given period of time, it reaches an upper threshold of pressure. When that upper threshold is reached, the production of cerebrospinal fluid is turned off by a home-ostatic mechanism. When a lower threshold of pressure is reached, production is turned on again. In this manner a rhythmic rise and fall of fluid pressure is achieved. This, in turn, causes the rhythmic changes in the boundaries of what constitutes a semi-closed hydraulic system. That is, a synchronous rhythmic movement is imparted to the cranium, dura mater, sacrum, fascia, and virtually every aspect of the body.

CranioSacral Therapists use the palpation of the craniosacral rhythm to locate restrictions in the system, and they have a sequence of sensitive methods for releasing them. The practice of CST is an art as well as a science. Its effectiveness depends upon the sensitivity of practitioners and their capacity to listen intimately to what the cranio-sacral pulse is saying, and then to respond intuitively—based on knowledge, experience and training—to the minute particulars of the individual client's condition at the precise moment of the treatment. The basic method involves coaxing the craniosacral system to find its own way back to regular functioning.

Techniques for Modifying Craniosacral Rhythm

As I say, we coax the craniosacral system, we do not force it. When the therapist detects an irregularity or restriction, he or she attempts to prevent the craniosacral rhythm from returning via that abnormal position by encouraging it to find a new route. Such coaxed discov-ery of new routes introduces added mobility into the system and its library of motions.

The craniosacral system actually has its own natural way of cor-recting restrictions and irregularities. This is the "still point," a con-dition lasting from a few seconds to a few minutes during which the craniosacral rhythm comes to a halt. The therapist often attempts to help the system arrive at a still point. This is called "still point induction." Still points can be induced from various places on the body.

One method is through the feet. The therapist cradles the heels in his or her hands, tuning in to the external rotation (flexion phase), the return to neutral, the excursion into internal rotation (extension phase), and so on. Say the left foot rotates externally further than the right, and that neither rotates internally as easily as it does externally. In order to change this less-than-perfect situation, the therapist follows the motion of each foot to the furthest point to which it moves with the greatest ease. In our example this would mean that the therapist follows both feet into external rotation. At this point he or she resists the return to neutral by making his or her hands immobile. The therapist does not push further into external rotation; the return is simply resisted. The rest of the system will return to neutral and go into internal rotation, but with less facilitation. As the therapist observes this movement, he or she takes up the slack in the movement and follows it—just as you would keep the front bumper of your automobile snug against the rear bumper of a car you were pushing. If this process of resisting and then taking up slack is repeated a number of times, the feet will rotate a little further each time. Eventually the total craniosacral system will "shut down," i.e., become perfectly still. This is the still point.

The still point is usually heralded by gross irregularities in the craniosacral motion. The system may shudder, pulsate or wobble. As the still point becomes imminent, the subject will often experience either an exacerbation of existing pain or the recurrence of an old familiar pain that is currently quiescent. The subject will also experience changes in breathing patterns and probably some light perspiration. During the still point itself, however, everything relaxes. The pain disappears. Breathing becomes very easy. Muscle tension melts away. When the still point is over, the craniosacral system resumes its motion, usually with better symmetry and larger amplitude.

Induction of still point at the head or sacrum is usually effected more rapidly than at the feet, but it requires greater sensitivity. The

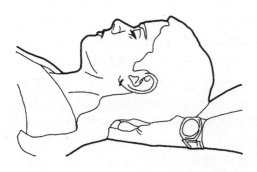
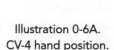
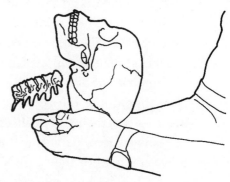

Illustration 0-6A.
CV-4 hand position.

Illustration 0-6B.
CV-4 relationship to bony structures.

technique for inducing a still point at the head is called the CV-4. [See Illustrations 0-6 A and B.] This produces a slight compression of the 4th ventricle of the brain. The head of the client is held in the facilitator's hands. Widening of the head is resisted; no pressure is applied by the therapist. The craniosacral system of the client furnishes the force; the therapist simply resists that force. This increases the fluid pressure within the cranium and causes it to be redirected along all other available pathways. The CV-4 technique promotes fluid movement and exchange. It affects diaphragm activity and respiration, and seems to relax the sympathetic nervous system to a significant degree. I have often used this technique to reduce tension in stressed patients. Improvement of the functioning of the autonomic nervous system (the aspect of the nervous system that regulates physiological processes) is always expected as a result of still point induction.

Basic Principles and Range of Application

CranioSacral Therapy is based on the discovery of the concrete physiological facts, processes and techniques I have outlined above; its effectiveness, however, depends on much more than the mastery of anatomical and physiological information and the ability to perform its technical procedures. The subjective relationship between the therapist and client is enormously important. I would like to conclude this introduction by mentioning some of the more general principles of CranioSacral Therapy and how they affect this relationship. I will also provide some idea of the range of problems it can help to alleviate.

For CranioSacral Therapy to work properly, the therapist must trust that all the information necessary to understand the underlying causes of a client's health problems, as well as what must be done to resolve them, lie within the client. It thus becomes the responsibility and goal of the CranioSacral Therapist from the beginning to establish a working rapport with this well of information and understanding. In CranioSacral Therapy and the practices that grew out of it, such as SomatoEmotional Release, this information itself becomes available through what I came to call the "Inner Physician." The Inner Physician is the aspect of the client's being that knows all about his or her condition. The skilled CranioSacral Therapist is able to contact and elicit the Inner Physician's cooperation in the therapeutic process. In the main text of this book I hope it will become clear how the Inner Physician participates in the healing work.

In order to develop rapport, the therapist must impart to the client's Inner Physician that his or her intentions are to help deal with primary problems, not to mask core issues by offering symptomatic relief. Deep problems must be defined and resolved. The Inner Physician knows this and will not settle for less. If one set of symptoms is "cured" but a deeper problem is not resolved, this deeper problem may find another set of symptoms to present. It is as though the symptoms are a call for help from deep inside the client. Core problems may be physical, emotional and/or spiritual. The CranioSacral Therapist must establish a relationship with the Inner Physician in order to help the client get to this problem. When the deeper problem is resolved, the symptoms dissolve with perhaps just a little help from the therapist.

It is, of course, not true that all symptoms have deep underlying causes. Some are simply happenings that occur. But in CranioSacral Therapy we believe that every symptom, pain or complaint deserves an investigation to determine whether or not it is the voice of a deeper problem or simply something such as a freak accident, an infection, etc. The Inner Physician knows the answer to this question and will share it willingly with the therapist once a trusting relationship has been established.

Initially, CranioSacral Therapy employs a soft, gentle use of the hands to facilitate the self-correction of the craniosacral system. This touch is concurrently used to convey to the Inner Physician the love, trust and sincere dedication of the therapist. This loving, trusting and dedicated energy is offered without conditions or strings attached in order to facilitate the deepest possible healing.

Once this trust is established, the CranioSacral Therapist must also trust the information received from the client's body and the Inner Physician; otherwise, the information will stop coming. It is as though the Inner Physician rejects the therapist. In such cases the therapist will be able to do superficial structural work with the craniosacral system, but probably will not be able to get to deep problems until the trust is developed.

I do not believe that CranioSacral Therapists should think of particular symptoms as always following from the same causes in a one-two fashion. Each client, and even each occurrence of a symptom in a client, is an individual case. Expectations that the same symptom always, or even often, derives from the same cause can be very misleading, especially when the therapist is relying upon very subtle body-motion signals as is the case in the use of CranioSacral Therapy. These signals may be merely imagined by the therapist if he or she expects to find them. It is better to not even know the client's complaint when the body evaluation is done. When I begin a session with a patient I have seen before, I try not to remember what I found out previously. I always evaluate the situation freshly at the beginning of each session. I may find new developments that might otherwise escape me if I already have a mindset when I re-evaluate. After the initial evaluation for each session there is plenty of time to integrate previous findings with the patient's report of changes, new pains, etc.

This last point is exceedingly important, though it goes against the grain of most medicine as it is conventionally practiced. The following story will illustrate, I think poignantly, what I am talking about.

In 1966 I was in practice in Clearwater Beach, Florida. One evening I was called to make a motel house call. It was about 9:00 P.M. when I arrived. A woman was lying on her bed with a very severe headache. Her husband presented me with a letter from a doctor at a highly reputable medical clinic in the north. The letter stated that his patient suffered from severe migraine headaches. It suggested that the treatment of choice would be an injection of fifty to seventy-five milligrams of the powerful synthetic narcotic Demerol. Upon examining her, I began to suspect she had a brain tumor rather than a migraine headache. I gave her the Demerol for her pain after I completed my examination, which took three or four minutes. The shot helped a little.

I tried to convince her husband that he should let me hospitalize her. He finally agreed and we went to the hospital by ambulance. She died during the night. The autopsy revealed that she had malignant brain tumors. Perhaps she originally had been a victim of migraines. But failure to re-evaluate each episode afresh may have cost her her life. I decided at the time not to accept previous diagnoses from medical clinics, no matter how reputable the facility.

There is virtually no limit to the kinds of problems CranioSacral Therapy might help to alleviate. CranioSacral Therapy always improves fluid movement in all systems throughout the body. By doing this it enhances many functions: the provision of nutrients to cells; the removal of toxins and waste products from the tissues; the circulation of immune cells, thereby increasing the body's natural defenses against disease-producing bacteria and viruses; the delivery of fresh blood to organs and tissues; and the movement of cerebrospinal fluid. Thus, the only situations in which CranioSacral Therapy should not be applied are those in which the above results are undesirable for some reason.

We are now ready to look at SomatoEmotional Release: its definition, its history and its practice.

Chapter One

The Evolution of a Concept

Definition

SomatoEmotional Release (SER) is the expression of emotion that, for reasons deemed appropriate by some part of a person's nonconscious, has been retained, suppressed and isolated within the soma. The word "soma" is Greek for "body." For our purposes we might think of the soma as the body psyche. Observation of the SER process suggests that independent retention of the energy or memory of both physical and emotional trauma is frequently accomplished by specific body parts, regions and viscera.

The SER process is initiated by hands-on communication between the therapeutic facilitator and the client. It is the result of meaningful and intentioned touch. The meaning and intention of the touch may be either conscious or nonconscious.

Psychiatrists and psychotherapists who have witnessed or participated in the SER process often liken it to body psychotherapy. In this analogy we see the client's body movements as analogous to the verbal aspect of psychotherapy. From clinical observation it would appear that most somatically retained trauma and emotion originally occurred against a background dominated by physiologically destructive emotions such as anger, fear or guilt. This destructive emotional background may have been specific to the moment of the traumatic event or a more generally negative state of mind.

Personal observation and participation in hundreds of SER processes

---

The Nonconscious

The word "nonconscious" is used throughout this book to denote any bodily, mental, or spiritual process or situation not within the patient's conscious awareness at the time under discussion. The word was coined to avoid the wide variety of connotations—correct or incorrect—which have accumulated around the words "unconscious" and "subconscious." The nonconscious refers to any part of us—from the highest self to the lowest aspect of our being—of which we are unaware.

---

has led me to postulate that organs, tissues, and perhaps individual cells possess memory, emotional capacity and intellect. Release of retained tissue emotion and pain usually passes through the client's conscious awareness either at the time of the SER experience or within twenty-four to forty-eight hours. Conscious recall of past incidents connected to tissue memories most frequently occurs as a sudden insight within a few hours, if not at the time, of SER. It is not uncommon for clients to consciously experience tissue-related emotion at the time of SER and to have recall of the original incident later.

The Discovery of SomatoEmotional Release

The concept of SomatoEmotional Release did not arise from purely intellectual considerations. It came as the result of clinical experiences under various circumstances that all began to point toward the same central focus.

In the late 1970s I was a principal investigator in research at a county center for autism in Genessee County, Michigan. We aimed our work at the possible use of CranioSacral Therapy in the treatment of autism. At the same time, I was working with Dr. Zvi Karni, a biophysicist and bioengineer on loan to our department at Michigan State University from the Technion Institute at Haifa, Israel. Dr. Karni and I were investigating and successfully measuring the effects of my therapeutically intended touch and manipulative procedures upon the baseline electrical potential of the human body. I was concurrently seeing private patients outside these research settings.

Research With Autistic Children

The first year of our work with autistic children focused on observations of their characteristic behaviors and personalities, as well as physical examinations and craniosacral and structural evaluations. We also conducted blood, urine and hair analyses. There were twenty-six children in our research project. We studied the children's responses to our attempts to move into their private worlds—worlds that were, at least on the surface, very isolated.

We observed that gentle, non-intrusive, well-intentioned touch was the most acceptable entry. We also discovered that still point induction by the use of this accepted gentle touch helped us to establish a positive rapport with the autistic child. Our team was made up of myself, Dianne L. Upledger (my wife) and Jon D. Vredevoogd, as well as an ever-changing stream of interested and dedicated graduate students. Some of these students were from the Osteopathic College at Michigan State University and some were from related healthcare colleges. We all did hands-on work and began to appreciate and know the value and potential of well-intentioned touch.

During the second year of this research project, we began exploring various therapeutic approaches. We used nutritional counseling with parents and guardians. We modified the physical environment in terms of lighting, temperature and humidity. We used ten percent CO_2/ninety percent O_2 inhalation therapy to stimulate deeper breathing. We used a variety of indicated manual therapies for structural mobilization and corrections. And last, but not least, we applied CranioSacral Therapy once a week to each child.

Over the years it has become clear to me that I can learn much more by observing than I can by invading. This was not always true of my approach. During my first ten years in private general practice and emergency room coverage, I was an invader par excellence. "Make it happen" was my motto. Fortunately, I tempered that attitude to some extent, and I became ninety percent observer and ten percent invader in our craniosacral work with autistic children.

The progression of events with most autistic children in our research project went something like this: First, the establishment of rapport and trust was imperative. We did this patiently and quietly, first by touch and then by the induction of still points wherever our hands were touching the child. We frequently induced still points at the knees, shoulders, feet, or arms. We seldom were able to work from the head for the first several sessions, since they often took place on the floor under the treatment table. We worked wherever the children wanted to be and wherever they would allow us to touch their bodies. Sometimes an autistic child would allow only one of us at a time to touch him; almost without exception, however, three or four of us would eventually be able to touch the child at the same time.

Not infrequently these autistic children would object violently to the touch of one of us but allow touch from another. This response made us aware of the power of the "toucher's" intention and how it is nonconsciously or consciously broadcast to the "touchee." When, on occasion, I sensed negativity in a graduate student, I excluded that student from touching until a positive attitude was generated. I also had to occasionally excuse from the treatment room an assistant with a negative attitude. The autistic children clearly could discern the therapist/facilitator's intent and attitude. I'm sure that on some level they also understood the effect that attitude and intent might have upon their being.

My conversations with research physicist Neil Mohon have suggested that each of us has multiple and qualitatively different energy fields. Mohon's research using energy field detection devices has led him to believe that each human being may have as many as fifty different personal energy fields. Since energies may either attract or repel, he suggests that the most successful therapist/facilitators have energy fields that are attractive to a greater proportion of people. That is, the successful therapeutic facilitator's energy field has the least repellent potential. We know that sensitive organisms such as pet beagles will

Therapist/Facilitator and Therapeutic Facilitator

I have developed the combined terms "therapist/facilitator" and "therapeutic facilitator" to emphasize the correct approach to SomatoEmotional Release and its derivatives. They remind us that CranioSacral Therapy practitioners are essentially facilitating the inherent healing capacities and processes of the client. The therapist/facilitator accepts the concepts that each client is unique, that their problems are individual and unique, and that there is wisdom inside every one of them that understands each problem in terms of where it came from, whether or not it has a deeper purpose, and how it might best be resolved. The CranioSacral Therapy practitioner's role is to blend with that internal wisdom and *facilitate* its recommended processes.

automatically be attracted to or withdraw from certain individuals. This may be due to the nature of the projected energy. Autistic children may possess the same sensitivity. I believe, and Mohon agrees, that once therapeutic facilitators are aware of their energy field potential, they can modify it by intention or thought projection.

After the successful induction of still points during several visits, the autistic children usually became cooperative and assumed a supine position of their own volition upon the treatment table. I would then proceed to work with the child's head very gently and tenderly. Because focus is so important, I always concentrated on loving that child at that time. I would slowly add my assistants to the therapeutic session by having each one hold an individual upper or lower limb. Ultimately five of us usually treated a single cooperating autistic child during each CranioSacral Therapy session. Most sessions lasted for twenty minutes. Today I feel that longer and more frequent Cranio-Sacral Therapy sessions would have produced much more dramatic results, but we were working under rather inflexible time constraints.

As we treated each child it seemed that, after a few preliminary cranial vault releases, we always encountered a severe restriction of the floor of the cranial vault. It was while working with these children that I began to more fully appreciate how many kinds of restrictions can arise at the cranial sutures. They all had to be released before the floor of the vault could be successfully decompressed.

Almost immediately a great reduction or total cessation of self-abusive and self-destructive behavior occurred in these decompressed children. By this I mean that the children voluntarily stopped banging their heads against the wall; or they stopped biting their wrists or hands; or they stopped gouging some favorite part of their body. It was as though the reason for self-inflicting pain no longer existed.

One can develop several viable hypotheses for this dramatic behavioral change. The most attractive hypothesis to me is that the compressed and restricted cranial bases of such children cause a deep, out-of-control pain inside their heads. Head banging and thumb pressure on the roof of the mouth—which was often mistakenly interpreted as thumb sucking—could be instinctive attempts to release the cranial base restrictions. Chewing on the wrist and otherwise gouging the flesh were, perhaps, attempts at either inducing elevated endorphin production, closing the "pain gate," or substituting a controllable pain for an uncontrollable pain. Perhaps a combination of these possibilities was in effect.

After—and only after—the successful front-to-back decompression of the floor of the cranial vault and the reduction or total cessation of self-abusive behavior did the next most remarkable and instructive phenomenon occur. After the release of the compression, it became apparent that there was severe side-to-side compression of some of the bones of the cranium itself. It was through our attempt to decompress these bones that two very useful happenings occurred. First, we devised the "Ear Pull" technique for decompression of the temporal bones. This is a method of mobilizing the temporal bones of the cranium by gently pulling on the ears. Second, and most significant to the origin of the concept of SomatoEmotional Release, the child's body began to move autonomously; that is, an arm or leg would show a tendency to move as though it had a mind of its own. We decided to follow these movements rather than try to inhibit them.

I was usually working with four assistants, one on each arm and one on each leg. During the times that these spontaneous body movements were occurring, the decompression of the temporal bones seemed impossible. This was why I began to pull gently on the ears. It made good sense to me because the ear is attached by connective tissue to the temporal bone.

I was unsuccessful in decompressing the temporal bones initially, but as we continued to work and gently try for temporal decompression, the amount of patient-induced limb and body movement continued to increase. This was not conscious, voluntary movement; it seemed automatic. By this stage of the treatment process the autistic child was typically in a deep state of relaxation, and the body was very loose and relaxed except for the subtle movement tendencies just described. These subtle movements occurred only when one of us held the involved body part. They usually began with a limb and then slowly spread to involve the torso, neck and head. As we followed, we became extremely sensitive to intended body movement. Without our following and lending physical support, the movement stopped. It was as though the therapeutic facilitator's touch imparted the energy necessary to initiate the body movement process. The continuation of the process depended heavily upon our ability to follow the most subtle body intentions, counteracting the forces of gravity without leading or inhibiting the child's body movement. As our skills developed, the body movements of these autistic children went further and further until they reached a position that seemed to be an apparent end point, a place where everything became quiet and still. It is this position that we later named the "therapeutic position." This end position could be either anatomically normal or quite abnormal.

I remember a child's right foot pointing directly backwards. It was rotated about one hundred and eighty degrees at its end point. He went into this position of his own volition and stated when questioned that he was very comfortable with it. (Later, after the Cranio-Sacral Therapy session, he could not achieve this anatomical position and would not allow us to put him into it.) As we waited at this point—

because we didn't know what else to do—there came a palpable release throughout the body. It was as though his body had opened. As muscles softened, fascia and connective tissues lengthened. And as fluids and energies began to flow more freely, the child cried. It was at these end points, while we were waiting, that total body release occurred.

We saw varying responses as we worked on these children. Some cried softly or wailed very loudly. Others expressed what looked like fear, anger and frustration. These expressions, both facial and postural, often continued for several minutes as body releases processed. When the releasing process was nearing completion, their facial expressions typically became more peaceful and loving. Once initiated, these events seemed to occur with each child more than once during a visit. In subsequent sessions the releases seemed progressively less intense, until finally no more spontaneous body motions occurred. Then and only then could I successfully decompress the temporal bones. I still cannot give a plausible explanation for the relationship between that specific restriction and the release of body tension and emotion we observed.

Inability to express love and hold affection for other humans is a hallmark of autism. After the releases of both body tension and emotional expression, these autistic children typically began to express affection toward other human beings. Another hallmark of autism is withdrawal from social contact. Following the releases, these children demonstrated sociable behavior and began to play with classmates.

We didn't know it at the time, but we had witnessed and participated in our introduction to SomatoEmotional Release.

The Use of Bioelectrical Measurements

While the research project on autism was under way, I worked independently with Dr. Karni in measuring potential electrical changes in the clients' bodies to see if they might correlate with various therapeutic activities. We investigated the effects of acupuncture, various types of osteopathic manipulation, and what was later named Cranio-Sacral Therapy on these electrical potentials.

We had begun our joint project as adversaries. With only a few months' seniority as a research clinician in the Department of Biomechanics, I had extended an open challenge to Dr. Karni and the department's five clinicians and twenty-two Ph.D. researchers. For years, I and other clinicians had subjectively perceived a transference of energy between ourselves and clients while we rested our hands on them for thirty seconds or more without performing any gross movements. The charge to the department was to use interdisciplinary means to investigate and measure these previously unexplained observations.

We had weekly Wednesday morning meetings chaired by an expert in experimental design. The disciplines represented by the Ph.D. group ranged from anatomy to psychology to biophysics. It was in this setting that I suggested we try to measure an exchange of energy between client and therapeutic facilitator during a hands-on treatment session. At first I was politely refused; later, the refusal was not so polite! I persisted in the presentation of this possible focus for research and was ultimately made a source of laughter. I didn't take kindly to being laughed at and became adamant, suggesting that perhaps the problem was too difficult for these physicists and engineers to tackle. This approach got a response from Dr. Karni, who agreed to work with me long enough to prove that, at least on this question, I was a crazy imbecile with delusions of grandeur. We began.

Dr. Karni first came in simply as an observer while I was seeing clinic patients. Since I was viewed as a specialist in biomechanics, most of my clinic patients were people suffering from long-standing pain. We normally thought that such pain was neuromusculoskeletal in origin and most often related to some sort of injury or trauma. Dr. Karni called to my attention that most of my treatments consisted of placing a patient's body or body part in a position that diminished or eliminated the patient's subjective sensation of pain. I usually held the patient in this position until certain cues indicated that the effect was complete. I would then reposition the patient's body and determine

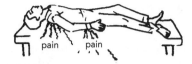

A. Patient in pain.

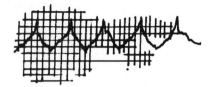

Electrical potential (during pain.)

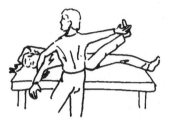

B. Patient's body moves into therapeutic position. Craniosacral rhythm stops. Facilitator holds therapeutic position until craniosacral rhythm begins again.

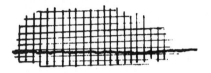

Electrical potential while craniosacral rhythm is shut down.

C. Craniosacral rhythm begins ... body is allowed to move to any position it indicates ... processes of "B" are repeated as necessary.

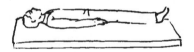

D. Pain is gone. Body returns to "normal" position.

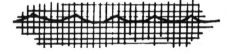

Electrical potential activity is soft and regular.

Illustration 1-1.
Correlations between body positions, electrical phenomena and subjective pain relief.

whether any direct technique should be carried out to mobilize an immobilized and "stuck" joint. More often than not, after repositioning the patient, nothing further was necessary.

After several hours of observation and rather agonizing question-and-answer sessions between Dr. Karni and me (it is difficult when you realize how little of what you do can be explained), we decided to consider the measurement of electrical potential inside the body. This approach assumed that the body is basically a skin-enclosed bag of electrically conductive fluids and tissues. (Later we would view the fascia as a specialized micro-conduction system within the skin.) In this model the skin acts as an insulator between what is inside of it and what is outside. We conveniently considered the skin acupuncture points as valves that would permit the flow of electrical energy to pass in or out in a controlled manner. On occasion these valves needed adjustment with needles or other methods of external stimulation. We did not hypothesize that the purpose of acupuncture points was necessarily to conduct electrical energy through the skin; it did and still does seem reasonable to me, nonetheless, that this is the function of some of these points.

We viewed the skin as the insulator barrier that maintains a differential in electrical potential between the constituents of the body it encloses and the external environment. In measuring electrical potential, the electrical "noise" produced by the muscle tissue is normally tuned out. We found, however, that the measurement of the amount of noise itself was a useful indicator; that is, the noise of electrical activity was high until we reached the body position that offered subjective pain relief to the patient. At this point in the treatment process, the electrical noise abruptly diminished and the baseline of electric activity moved toward zero on the polygraph tracing. It remained smooth and near zero as the "tissue release" progressed.

As we moved away from the therapeutic position, the baseline of the electrical potential moved away a little from the zero line, and some noiselike electrical activity returned. This noise was seldom as it was before we found the therapeutic position and obtained relief from pain.

After what seemed like a tremendous amount of work, observation, badgering, argument, and discussion, I was finally forced by Dr. Karni to realize that I nonconsciously relied on a certain physiological cue for discovering the position in which a patient would experience relief from pain. That cue was the sudden cessation of the craniosacral rhythm. After a brief interval, as the craniosacral rhythm began to return, I would sense the tissues relax, a release of heat from the body part I was holding, and the flow of fluid and energy. As these subtle phenomena occurred, I would reposition the body in a way that seemed comfortable and appropriate for that individual.

We observed this sequence of events on several occasions as the body position, subjective pain and changes in electrical, inside-the-skin phenomena occurred in concert. We played a lot of games with each other to test the interdependence of these variables. Without any cue from me, Dr. Karni would mark on the polygraph tracing when he thought I had found the right position for the therapeutic release. He set up a screen with he and his polygraph on one side and my patients and I on the other. He could not see what I was doing and I could not see him or his tracings. Dr. Karni developed the ability to view the tracings and tell me what I was feeling and doing with the patient. He also could accurately tell the patient when subjective pain relief occurred. Thus we continued. By now we were friends. We didn't know what we had stumbled onto, but we both were excited.

The polygraph tracings allowed us to see the levels of electrical potential inside the skin to a fraction of a millivolt. We could see the changes in electrical potential that occurred when the craniosacral rhythm stopped. We could see from the electrical potential when pain relief occurred. The electrical potential could thus tell us how long the therapeutic facilitator should maintain the specific therapeutic position that seemed to offer pain relief.

The next big question loomed unavoidably: Why should a specific body position relieve a situation that had begun several years before and had been symptomatically troublesome for a long time? Not far behind were other questions: By what mechanism does the craniosacral rhythm abruptly stop when we obtain the therapeutic position? How and why do the electrical potentials change in relation to these phenomena?

We decided to work on the big question of body position and pain relief first. It was the pursuit of the answer to this question that led us to the concept of energy cysts that we teach today.

Energy Cysts: A Model Is Suggested

As I mentioned, Dr. Karni forced me to realize that somehow I was helping the patient's body reach a position, contorted or otherwise, that offered pain relief. More often than not, the relief was permanent. How did this come about? Observation indicated that in the correct position—and it had to be correct to the millimeter—pain relief was accompanied by the softening of tissue and the relaxation of the whole body. It also produced a reduction of the respiratory rate, a palpable increase in fluid and energy flow through the involved body parts, and a release of heat. It is obvious why we came to call this correct position the therapeutic position. In each case the craniosacral rhythm stopped and changes in electrical potential occurred when we found this position. We wanted to know why a given, precisely correct body position made all this happen.

Dr. Karni directed me to the work of Erwin Schrödinger, the great German physicist of the first half of the 20th century who was one of the founders of quantum physics. Dr. Schrödinger is largely responsible for the concepts of entropy and negentropy (information). Our discussions led us to the idea that a traumatic injury is, in physical terms, an injection of energy into the victim's body. This would happen, for example, from a blow to the base of the spine when a fall is suddenly interrupted by a stair step. The stair step also suffers a blow from the base of the spine, but the stair step is itself immobile, and the energy of the impact simply passes through it. As we will see, something quite different happens to the tissue at the base of the spine. Another example is a blow to the head dealt by a hammer at the hands of a mugger.

In both of the above examples, energy is injected into the victim's body: in the first case by the stationary stair step and in the second by the moving hammer in the hand of the mugger. The quantity of energy and the energy's forward momentum as it enters the recipient's body are counterbalanced by the dampening effect of the body tissues the

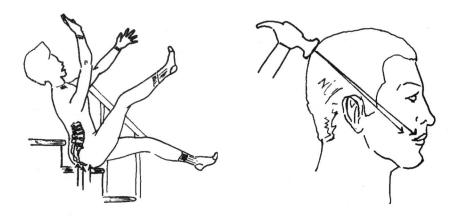

Illustration 1-2.
Arrows indicate direction and penetration of force vectors as they enter the body
during a traumatic experience. See text.

energy penetrates. This dampening effect relates to the viscosity or density of the tissues in the traumatic energy's path. If there were no dampening effect, the energy of the injury would simply go right through the victim's body and come out the other side. This does not happen. Body tissues have density and therefore provide a dampening effect that the momentum-driven injury force must penetrate. The distance of penetration is the result of the relationship between the quantity of force, its momentum, and tissue density. This can be expressed by the following formula in which K is a constant that converts this equation from qualitative to quantitative:

$$\frac{\text{Traumatic Force}}{\text{Tissue Density}} \times K = \text{Distance of Penetration}$$

The energy imparted by the victim's collision with the stationary stair step or with the hammer will penetrate into each body a given distance. This distance of penetration is proportional to the amount of force in the blow and is dependent upon the types of tissues it must penetrate—that is, the greater the force, the deeper the penetration;

the more dense the tissue, the greater the resistance to penetration. Where the energy of the injury stops is calculated by the above equation. Keep in mind that, for practical purposes, this energy of injury penetrates the body in a straight-line trajectory; it does not go around corners. However, energy also is bundled in "quantum parcels," so the energy actually gets divided into precisely discrete packages, as it were. In addition, the body itself will be in motion during the collision.

For example, say the actual impact of the collision took one-fifth of a second and the energy of injury entering the body divided into quantum parcels of one one-hundredth of a second each. Due to the body's motion from the impact of the injury, we would have twenty parcels of energy entering the body, each with its own straight-line trajectory, adding up to the one-fifth of a second during which the collisional forces were operative. The body's inertial resistance to being moved would cause it to begin its movement response to the injury force after five one-hundredths of a second and continue moving throughout the duration of the collision. This would mean that the first five parcels of energy would share the same straight line of energy trajectory, while each of the subsequent fifteen energy parcels would have independent and slightly different trajectories.

As a body moves in response to a collision, the movement causes each previous straight-line trajectory to become bent. The next energy parcel makes its own new straight-line trajectory, and this in turn is bent and rendered obsolete by the body's continuing motion response. Our model requires that the trajectory path of traumatic force entry must be straight in order for the injury energy to exit the body the same way it went in. If the trajectory path of entry is bent, the injury energy is trapped at the end of its penetration.

Once this energy enters the recipient's body, it must be dealt with. It is an abnormal input of excess energy. It is disruptive to the controlled, functioning energy systems of the body. As I mentioned previously, Dr. Karni and I conceived of the human body as a skin-enclosed bag of electrical conductors having various degrees of conductivity. We envisioned the body fluids as very conductive, and we saw the

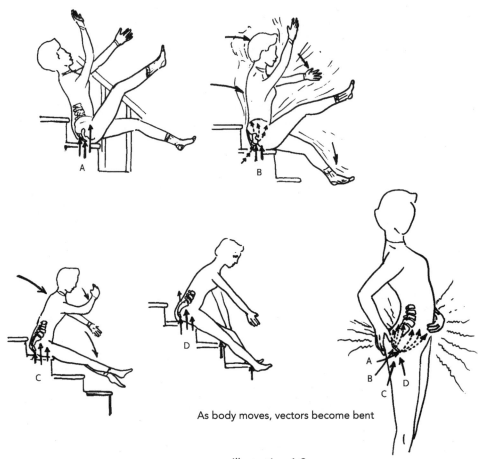

Illustration 1-3.
Arrows demonstrate bending of force vectors (entry trajectories) as body position changes during the duration of impact with the step. This creates multiple energy cysts at different locations. See text.

connective tissues as possessing specific properties of conduction for micro-currents that somehow nurture these tissues. (We also saw acupuncture meridians as specialized lines of conductivity within the tissues.) This model begins to suggest the existence of specialized conductive qualities present in specific conductor tissues that match certain electrically energetic systems.

We reasoned that the energy of injury penetrates the body tissues

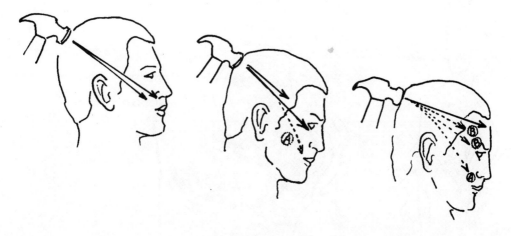

Illustration 1-4.
Hammer blow to the head introduces vectors as described in text. Trajectories are
bent as head moves in response to the blow.

to the appropriate depth at which the body must determine what to
do with these parcels of unwanted energy. As far as the body is concerned, this externally derived energy is disorganized and chaotic. It
does not fit into the bodily organization of the intrinsic energy systems. The unwanted energy may lodge in such organs as the brain,
intestines or heart. Once there, it can disrupt visceral function or
lodge in the connective tissues, bones or joints, causing pain as well
as dysfunction. Wherever it lodges it will disrupt efficient function.
The body's first choice is to dissipate this disruptive energy. The next
best choice is to localize it. When localized, it creates problems in
the smallest area possible. The intrinsic energy systems must then
work around this localized area of disorganized energy. This accom-
modation of the extrinsic disorganized energy comes at some cost to
the victim's body, but the expenditure is necessary.

Dr. Karni and I thought of the localized area of extrinsic, disorganized energy as an area of increased entropy, as described by Erwin
Schrödinger in the 1930s. Dr. Schrödinger hypothesized that entropy
can be reorganized by intelligent means in biological systems. He
called this reorganization "information." In short, an unchecked

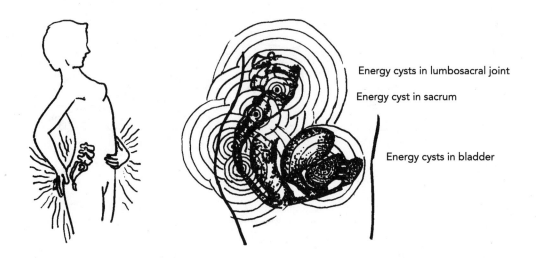

Illustration 1-5A.
Multiple locations of energy cysts. Each is best released via the body position
that provides a straight exit pathway for this energy. Thus, the body position of
entry must be mimicked.

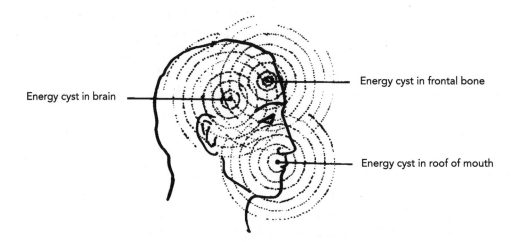

Illustration 1-5B.
Multiple locations of energy cysts in the head after the hammer blow.
Each is best released in the body position at the time of entry.
This makes the energy trajectories straight.

increase in entropy results in total disorganization, death and decomposition. Biological systems, however, can reverse or inhibit the increase in entropy by using information to cause a reorganization or release of this energy so that it can be used for the restoration of function within the system.

Dr. Karni suggested that I was reading the patient's body signals and assisting in the provision of information by attaining the therapeutic position that resulted in the release of the excess, highly entropic, disruptive energy. The release of this unwanted energy was analogous to the injection of information into a system of increasing entropy, resulting in improved function and remission of pain. As I described this conceptual model to the research staff at the Menninger Foundation in Topeka, Kansas, Dr. Elmer Green, the research director, raised his hand and said, "John, you have just described a cyst of energy." The name stuck.

Back to our model. It seemed reasonable that exact positioning of the connective tissue would align its fibers to enhance micro-current flow. This would allow the escape of disorganized or excess energy from the energy cysts to the exterior surface and then out of the body. We felt this phenomenon as heat during the release that occurred while in the therapeutic position. As we realigned the connective tissue fibers to improve conduction, we allowed entropy to decrease.

Dr. Karni used the example of a copper wire to help me understand what he thought was happening. As we know, copper is an excellent conductor of electricity. If we hit a copper wire with a hammer, we reduce its conductivity by disorganizing its particles. If we stretch the copper wire and realign the particles within it, we restore its full conductivity. [See Illustration 1-6.] Dr. Karni thought that a similar phenomenon could occur in connective tissue. That is, we could realign the fibers in the therapeutic position to allow improved conduction and the expulsion of unwanted external energy.

We then added to our model the idea that the most efficient escape route for the unwanted energy was its exact trajectory of entry. Each trajectory of entry had to be re-established to allow the release of its

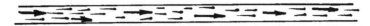

A. Copper wire with unimpaired electrical conduction

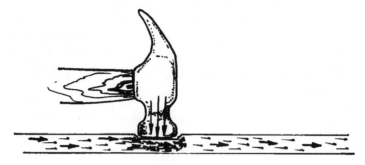

B. Impaired conduction of wire secondary to hammer blow

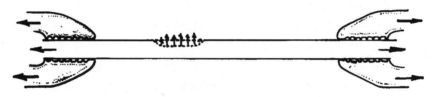

C. Tractioning [stretching] wire to normalize its structure

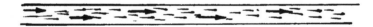

D. [Normal] electrical conductivity is restored

Illustration 1-6.
Demonstrates effect of hammer blow [B] and tractioning [C] of copper wire upon the wire's conductivity.

specific energy parcel in the reverse direction; therefore, several very closely related positions had to be found during a single session.

It appeared that each energy parcel had to be released along its own original entry pathway. Both the hypothetical stair step and hammer injuries described previously involved twenty parcels of energy.

Before the body overcame inertia and began to move in response to the collision, five parcels had entered the body from each impact. Then, after body movement began, each parcel of the last fifteen in the individual injuries had its own slightly different trajectory. Therefore, to obtain full therapeutic effect would require sixteen therapeutic body positions of release for each of the two injuries. It followed that there would be sixteen positions of the body around the base of the spine and sixteen positions of the head at which the craniosacral rhythm would stop. The electric potential baseline would drop and smooth out as all the other phenomena of release occurred. (The job of the therapeutic facilitator is to very sensitively follow the client's body movement tendencies, discover the therapeutic positions, and very patiently wait for the release phenomena to move to completion in each position.)

Another phenomenon that frequently accompanies the attainment of the therapeutic position is the expression of emotion related to the injury. There is frequently a re-experiencing of the injury by the client. It is as if the energy cyst holds the memory of its physical creation as well as the emotion that was present at that time. As the person becomes aware of the emotion and re-experiences it, the last effects of the energy cyst are removed completely. He or she can now view the whole incident in a symptom-free condition with a certain emotion-free, objective detachment.

For example, the client who slipped on the stairs and landed at the bottom on her "bottom" may have experienced fear, panic and anger about the slippery steps at the same time she realized she was falling. These same feelings would be felt during the release of the energy cysts.

Two other questions must be answered if this model is to hold up: What conditions favor the dissipation of the energy of injury, and what conditions favor its retention and the formation of an energy cyst?

Clinical observation led us to the concept that a background of destructive emotions, such as fear, anger or guilt, favors energy cyst formation, whereas a background of constructive emotions such as love and joy, favors dissipation followed by normal healing and rehabilitation. The destructive emotional background might or might not be related to the specific injury.

If a person falls off the stairs onto a concrete walkway while running out of the house in a very elated state of mind to greet a long-lost friend, and does not arouse enough fear or panic to overpower such happiness, the injury will probably heal without energy cyst formation. If, on the other hand, that person falls while running out of the house to escape the yelling of an irate spouse, the energy of injury will very likely penetrate and be retained as an energy cyst. The same would be true of our mugging victim. If he was in a good mood prior to the attack, and didn't see the hammer blow coming, he would suffer the immediate physical damage but probably not form an energy cyst. This does not mean there would not be significant brain damage and related dysfunction, but it does mean that the victim would reach maximal recovery without the complications of an energy cyst. If, however, the victim was worrying about the stock market crashing at the time of the hammer blow from the mugger, energy cyst retention would most likely occur.

Before discussing these complications, I would like to mention several other conditions that favor energy cyst formation. I have occasionally seen patients in good health and spirits whose injuries were so powerful that they overcame the person's ability to dissipate the energy. I have also seen energy cyst formation in good-spirited people who are in the recovery phase of a health problem. Such people may be physically unable to throw off the force of injury from a present physical trauma. The most common condition that favors energy cyst formation and retention, however, is the presence of related or unrelated destructive emotion at the time of injury.

Complications of Energy Cyst Retention

The complications deriving from energy cyst retention depend upon the cyst's emotional content, the quantity of energy within the cyst, and its location. It seems that the emotional content of an energy cyst is capable of entraining the general emotional tone of the whole person; that is, if the energy cyst is full of anger, self-righteous indignation and panic (as it might be with a mugging victim struck on the head in broad daylight in Middletown, U.S.A., where it was supposed to be perfectly safe), the victim's whole personality might change. He might become quick to anger and always feel justified in expressing it. The victim might also develop a phobia about strangers walking behind him. I have seen marked personality changes for the better occur after the release of an energy cyst that contained destructive emotion.

The physical and physiological effects of a retained energy cyst depend largely upon its potency (quantity of contained energy) and its location. For example, the energy from a fall on the base of the spine can penetrate quite easily into the organs in the pelvis. There it can cause bladder dysfunction with chronic sphincter-control problems, menstrual dysfunction, inability to conceive or maintain a pregnancy, prostatitis, and so on, depending upon the exact location of the energy cyst. If it doesn't penetrate to the viscera, pain in the tailbone is a good possibility. On the other hand, if it goes all the way to the respiratory diaphragm, the patient might later begin to notice symptoms of heartburn. If it goes through the diaphragm, it might penetrate into the heart and set the person up for coronary disease at a later date.

The energy cyst doesn't produce its full effect right away. The patient's body adapts as best it can; but slowly, over a period of months and years, the seat of the energy cyst is compromised in its function. By its presence, the energy cyst naturally contributes to the facilitation of the related spinal cord segments. The whole syndrome of segmental facilitation begins.

My work with Dr. Karni, our observations of the phenomena related to the energy cyst, and my work at the Center for Autism set the scene for the further clinical observations that I shall now describe.

Facilitated Segments

Usually the word "facilitated" has a positive connotation, implying that some process is made easier or more efficient. In the case of a "facilitated segment," however, it means that the stimulus threshold, i.e., the resistance to the conduction of an electrical impulse in a particular spinal cord "segment," has been reduced. This means that the facilitated segment of the spinal cord is excitable, and a smaller stimulus will trigger impulse firing in the segment.

This hypersensitivity may be detrimental to the body as a whole, depending on the tissues involved. For example, if the segment that provides nerves to the stomach becomes facilitated, the stomach becomes hypersensitive. The person who has this problem may be said to have a "nervous stomach" or to possess food allergies or intolerances. In fact, this problem will disappear if the facilitation is corrected.

A facilitated segment produces palpable changes in tissue texture. The muscles along the spine and connective tissue develop a "shoddy" feel, and joints in the area are less mobile. The tissues are tender to the touch and often painfully irritable. There are also changes in skin texture, sweat gland activity, and capillary supply to the skin.

Facilitated segments seem to occur at areas of focus for postural stress, sites of trauma, and segments of the spinal cord related to visceral problems. Once established, a facilitated segment can continue for years, even ultimately contributing to death. A facilitated segment at the fourth thoracic vertebra may cause decreased vitality of the heart, leading to blockage of coronary arteries and heart attack.

Therapeutically, any approach that interrupts the self-perpetuating activity of the facilitated segment will be helpful. CranioSacral Therapy is certainly one such approach in that it reduces activity in the sympathetic nervous system, reduces general stress and anxiety, helps endocrine function, assists in postural balancing, and improves fluid exchange.

Adapted from *CranioSacral Therapy II: Beyond the Dura*, pages 214–216

Observations in the Clinic

The following observations were made on private patients who were referred to me as a specialist in manual medicine, biomechanics and osteopathic manipulation techniques. While these individuals were not involved with us as research subjects, I shall nonetheless describe a few of these experiences to provide the flavor of what I was shown.

A thirty-eight-year-old professional woman divorced for almost ten years was referred to me by the Department of Psychiatry for consultation about possible structural musculoskeletal causes for persistent and severe pain in the low back and head. She had undergone a vaginal hysterectomy at age twenty-eight under duress from her then-husband. His insistence was based on the inconvenience tendered him by her PMS. In spite of her compliance, he divorced the patient within a year after the hysterectomy. She had been in psychotherapy for approximately seven of the ten years that had elapsed since the procedure. Subjects of concern in her psychotherapy included anger toward men in general, her condition of premature sterility, and the probability that the head and low back pain were psychosomatically induced.

During her first visit I found some somatic dysfunctions of the pelvis and neck. Osteopathic and craniosacral therapeutic techniques were applied, and she reported instant relief from pain. This kind of miraculous "cure" should make therapists suspicious once they come to grips with their own "therapist's ego." I had met my therapist's ego several years before and was very suspicious that this was only the beginning of my relationship as physician to this pain patient.

After approximately ten days the patient called and said that about fifty percent of her head and back pain had returned. She asked me to see her again. Our next session was about two weeks after the first. I treated her in a similar manner, but this time she did not experience the miraculous relief of pain that she did during the first office visit. She showed me her anger, and I knew that psychotherapy had not successfully resolved her negative feelings toward the male gender. She accused me of intentionally leaving her in pain because I secretly hated women. It was not a pleasant experience, but I had learned over the years not to take such accusations seriously. In any event, her anger didn't prevent her from insisting on seeing me again in a week's time.

In retrospect, it is obvious that I was encountering the conflict between what we now see as the part of the patient that wants Somato-Emotional Release—I didn't know what SER was at that time—and the part of her that resisted confrontation with the truth. I frequently view this latter part of the patient as the martyred part who says, "Leave well enough alone. I will protect you from this horrible memory realization. My happiness doesn't matter."

At the third visit, the patient reported a little improvement, probably enough to allow her to consciously justify another treatment session with me. Fortunately I had a graduate student observing during this visit. The patient was supine on the treatment table. I had my right hand under her left buttock with my fingers on the sacroiliac. With my left hand I was moving her left leg up and down gently to evaluate sacroiliac mobility and function. Quite suddenly her left leg flexed at the hip and knee. With no one touching it, the right leg did the same thing. I asked the graduate student to support her right leg gently while I did the same with her left.

This experience occurred during the period in which we were seeing emotional releases related to body positions at the Center for Autism. My intuition told me to manage her legs in a way that was similar to how we were obtaining emotional releases by body position with autistic children. Almost immediately after her legs reached the flexed position, we could see a lot of rapid eye movement going on beneath her closed lids. As luck would have it, her purse was in a chair that was within reach of her left hand.

The next thing I knew, she was pummeling my head, neck and right shoulder with her purse. I registered surprise and probably expressed some expletive—although I can't tell you exactly what that was. She quickly explained, as though she were a detached third-person observer, that the blows were meant for the surgical resident who was leaning too heavily on her left knee. His weight was creating a severe strain in her back and pelvis. She went on to explain that the anesthesiologist had her neck and head in an awkward position of extension that was very painful. She also said that all this happened during her hysterectomy and that she was completely asleep under the influence of anesthesia at the time.

I was taken a bit by surprise by this turn of events. I had done a fair amount of hypnoregression and hypnotherapy in the past and was aware that the nonconscious knows all or near all. I was no stranger to the idea that conversation and events during surgical procedures under general anesthesia might be recorded in the nonconscious mind. Yet all I had done was touch this lady at the left buttock and sacroiliac areas and passively move her left leg to test for sacroiliac mobility—and here she was visualizing her hysterectomy while asleep under a general anesthetic.

My first inclination was to let out an explosive "Wow!" I instead contained my enthusiasm and acted as if this was an everyday occurrence. I talked with her about how she shouldn't be mad at the surgical resident because he was probably exhausted from the hideously long hours required by the hospital during training. I tried my best to get her to empathize with him and to forgive and forget.

The anesthesiologist was more difficult to defend. He had been pulling on her head and was mightily straining and compressing her neck while the protective muscles were rendered essentially helpless by drugs. He had put a tube down her throat, made some remarks about how she was "keeping the playpen but losing the baby carriage," and was, in general, somewhat less than respectful. I tried to convince her that to stay angry with him, though it might be justified, was hurting her and not him. She accepted this idea to some extent, and her re-experiencing of the surgery ended by her choice just as quickly as it had begun.

I was convinced that we had discovered and dealt with the reasons for her acute anger at men. I thought I understood why the psycho-therapy had hit an impasse. I set another appointment for the following week. I really wanted to see what was going to happen. As it turned out, I was both over-enthusiastic and incorrect.

Her next visit was heralded by complaints of nervousness and an inability to concentrate, though her pains were appreciably improved. She had not seen her psychotherapist since her first visit with me, which made it about four weeks without psychotherapy. As she lay on the table in a supine position, the same graduate student was with me. (He had been totally astonished by the events of the last visit. I could not have prevented his attendance at this visit had I wanted to.) This time I made sure there were no potential weapons within her reach, and we brought her into the flexed-kneed position again. Today I would not be nearly so direct, but we were eager and had little idea of what we were actually onto as far as therapeutic approach was concerned. There were no ground rules yet.

She (her body) accepted our manual, non-verbal suggestions, and her legs went directly to the position as though she were in gynecological stirrups. Her head stretched autonomously on her neck into what appeared to be an uncomfortable position. She immediately began to describe the scene in the operating room as a third-party observer. She described in anatomical detail the dissection of tissues around her uterus as it was being removed through her vagina. She concurrently described and reacted in bodily ways to the sensations of tugging and pulling in her pelvis as the surgical procedure continued. Finally it was done. The uterus was put in a pan and sent to the pathology laboratory. She then related that the resident who had been leaning on her left leg was told to repair the vaginal incision. "Cuff" was the word she used. She felt this activity as the resident went about the repair process.

The surgeon paid little attention. He passed the time in conversation with the surgical nurse. When the resident finished closing the incision, the surgeon stepped back into the operating area, sat on a stool, looked at the resident's work, and remarked that it was a pretty sloppy job. He followed the remark with a statement to the effect that, if he had time, he would take those sutures out and make the resident do it over. The next case was ready, though, so he didn't have time.

The patient was furious. I tried to convince her that this castigation of residents and interns is a favorite sport among surgeons and other "hot shots," and that the repair was probably fine. She told me that, while this may be true, she had carried an incisional infection for about six months after the surgery and had healed very poorly. She felt that this was one of the things that had prompted her husband to divorce her. He had said that her inability to have satisfactory sex had driven him to seek satisfaction elsewhere. I tried to convince her that if this was all it had taken to break up her marriage, she was probably better off without the relationship. I also tried to convince her that the surgical repair might have been fine but that the non-consciously received suggestion that it was a second-rate repair might have been enough to slow down and complicate the healing process. (I only wanted to soften her anger.) What finally worked was the idea, once again, that being angry with her doctors from ten years ago was hurting her and not them. Anger is a destructive emotion when chronically produced and retained.

After just a few weeks of what I would now call "bodywork" and "ventilation," she was totally fine. She did not return to psychotherapy. She did, however, lecture to my students about her experiences. She had not had a relationship with a man since her divorce, but there was no rush; she was "desensitizing" [See page 131.]

The second case that crossed my path at about the same time was less dramatic but nearly as instructive as it unfolded. She was a twenty-seven-year-old single woman employed as a social worker in New York City. Her mother had been seeing me for chronic leg pain. The daughter had been referred by her mother. The daughter's problem was the gradual onset of increasingly debilitating pain of the left shoulder. I could find very little of a structural nature wrong with the shoulder joint, its related bones, the vertebral column, or the ribs.

I began the therapeutic positioning work. (This was the same work I was doing with Dr. Karni, but without electrical monitoring.) The patient's arm and shoulder went into a position that brought the craniosacral rhythm to an abrupt stop. I waited a few seconds, and movement of the arm, shoulder, neck, head, and total upper body began. The patient was sitting on the end of the table and I positioned myself to her left. She slowly began to lean way over to the left. Her craniosacral rhythm had not begun yet. She began to topple to her left as though she was going to fall to the floor onto her left shoulder. I managed to support her through this maneuver, allowing her to continue her slow descent toward the floor until her left shoulder was perhaps twelve or fourteen inches below the level of the table top. Her weight was supported by the table under her left hip and by me under her left shoulder. She stopped her movement here. My back was creaking, but she remained in this position for at least five minutes (it seemed like an hour) before her craniosacral rhythm began. When the rhythm began, she sat upright on the table, smiled, and told me she just realized that the shoulder problem was the result of a skiing injury when she was nineteen years old.

This single treatment session abated all her symptoms for about three months after she returned to New York. She then called and said that her shoulder didn't really hurt, but it was beginning to feel "funny" and become stiff.

She returned to my office in Michigan for two visits, one on a Friday and one on the following Monday. During the Friday visit I simply held her arm and head for awhile, but very little happened in the sitting position. I asked her to lie supine on the table and again held her left arm and shoulder. She moved a little, her craniosacral rhythm stopped, her shoulder became hot to the touch, and she suddenly felt very angry. I asked if she knew why she was angry. After a minute or two she said that the reason she had fallen while skiing was because another skier had cut in front of her. She had swerved as a reflexive, self-protective action and had fallen, injuring her left shoulder. She was angry with the skier who had cut in front of her. After telling me this, her craniosacral rhythm still did not start. I gently asked her if that was all she was mad about. She waited a few minutes, felt another strong surge of anger, and told me that what really made her mad was that the offending skier did not stop to see if she was all right or if she needed help. After she released this anger, she said she felt light and wonderful. On Monday she still felt fine. I gave her routine osteopathic and CranioSacral Therapy treatments.

I have seen her about every six months since then, simply because she likes the treatment process. She has had absolutely no further shoulder problems since the release of the anger, plus she has found herself better able to tolerate the frustrations of her profession as a social worker in New York City. (I'm sure her frustrations are many.)

Very soon after the surgical hysterectomy case, and between the first and second visits of the shoulder case, another surgical memory case came up. (I suppose this happened to properly impress me with the importance of the information to which I had become privy.) This case involved a woman in her mid-twenties who suffered from severe, debilitating headaches. I performed some routine CranioSacral Therapy techniques to loosen the various components of the cranial vault and the floor of the vault. Then I began the V-spread technique, which involves sending energy from one hand toward the other until you feel its arrival in the receiving hand.

As the V-spread energy began to build, the patient's craniosacral rhythm abruptly stopped. A lot of heat began to radiate from the area between her eyebrows. The patient began to feel a great deal of anger. This angry feeling calmed down as the heat radiation subsided and the V-spread seemed to take its full effect. The craniosacral rhythm recommenced its activity.

I asked the patient if she understood the anger that had expressed itself. She told me that it was hard for her to accept, but what came to mind was the surgeon operating on her nasal area some years before. As she re-experienced the surgical procedure, the surgeon seemed very angry. She had convinced him to put her to sleep for the surgery. He didn't like the idea but allowed a general anesthetic against his better judgment.

Here again we have an unconscious recording of an event during which the patient was supposed to be asleep. But this case poses other very fascinating questions. Does the emotion of the surgeon enter an energy cyst formed in the patient during the surgical procedure? Further, should we consider the surgical procedure a traumatic event able to produce an energy cyst? If so, does the anesthetized condition of the patient favor energy cyst formation and retention? The implications of these questions are immense.

SomatoEmotional Release

The experiences with autistic children, with Dr. Karni, and with the three patients just described came together simultaneously. It was as if these experiences had been orchestrated to tell me something. The unavoidable observation that surfaced was that the release of energy cysts leads to total-body releases that improve mind-body function. It further suggested that we do not need to know about the past injury. All we have to do is place our hands on the client in a gentle, sensitive manner; tune in to what the body wants to do; follow the movement; counter the effect of gravity; not lead the movement even if we think we know where it is going; and ask a few questions or give a little verbal support at critical times. The body will release not only energy cysts but the stored-up emotions that are contributing to patient discomfort.

With our hands we were releasing pent-up emotion via the somatic route. The demeanor and sociability of autistic children improved. Angry people became nicer. Pain went away. And the craniosacral rhythm stopped abruptly at the right time to tell us when we were on the right track. Who in the world would believe this? It worked, though, and the results were obvious.

During this fast-moving period, I began using Kirlian photography in my private practice. (See inset.) Using black-and-white Polaroid film, I took photos before and after each phase of a patient's treat-

---

Kirlian Photography

Kirlian photography is a technique for making photographs (without a camera) of the otherwise invisible patterns of energy that probably surround and permeate all material objects. Kirlian photography records the radiant energy around an object directly on photo-sensitive emulsion. The apparatus consists of a metal plate and an oscillator generating a high-voltage field of variable frequency. Placing the object on top of the metal plate, which is in contact with the emulsion, produces an image on the emulsion consisting of a luminous corona surrounding the object. The corona's characteristics vary with the object's energetic properties.

The Kirlian effect probably is caused by electrons emitted from the object that activate the photographic plate in the same way light does.

---

ment. The energy coronas projecting from both the patient's fingertips and mine markedly changed.

I had no real idea what I was onto, and it was more than a little awe-inspiring. It was also addictive. I was so intrigued I couldn't let go of it, and I didn't want to.

We needed a name for this process that would differentiate it clearly from psychosomatic medicine. It clearly wasn't the same, although it dealt with the body-mind interface. In a sense it was body-mind, not mind-body as was the psychosomatic concept. The name SomatoEmotional Release was coined.

I gathered up my courage and taught the first SomatoEmotional Release course in Chicago in 1980.

Chapter Two

Energy Cysts and SomatoEmotional Release

Energy Cysts and Arcing

The energy cyst is a localized area of increased entropy that is retained in the body. This increased entropy is disorganized and disruptive energy that the body handles the best way it can. Dr. Karni and I came up with the concept of the energy cyst based on our many observations of the bodily effects of externally induced trauma. This does not mean, however, that the only source of a localized area of increased entropy is an external physical trauma. It is simply that the sample that presented itself to us was composed of patients with physical residues that we named energy cysts.

The persistent question about energy cysts thus became whether they could be caused by means other than externally induced trauma; that is, could emotion, spiritual conflict, parasites, bacteria, viruses, toxins, malnutrition, or genetics induce an energy cyst?

I am now sure that areas of increased entropy or energy cysts can result from a wide range of problems. We must therefore specify the origin or cause of the energy cyst as accurately as we can. Is it induced emotionally, toxically, karmically, virally, or traumatically? Traumatically induced energy cysts are probably best released by finding and holding the correct therapeutic position. Other types of energy cysts can be released by the Direction of Energy technique, intention,

SomatoEmotional Release, and so on.

Energy cysts can be discovered in many ways. Occasionally it is as simple as letting the patient point to where it hurts, but I do not depend on this method. The patient may be experiencing a referred pain or secondary joint dysfunction. An energy cyst could also be obstructing energy flow anywhere along the course of an acupuncture meridian. The pain might then be felt in the related viscera or elsewhere along the meridian. You just can't depend on pain to show you where the energy cyst is located.

Arcing is probably the best method for localizing the energy cysts. Arcing is what I was doing intuitively when I evaluated and treated a patient—that is, until Dr. Karni forced me to try to describe it so that he could make good physics sense from my descriptions. After much observation and discussion, we decided that I was perceiving with my hands the energies that apparently emanate from an active lesion (a wound or an injury) that is really an energy cyst. We gave this the name "arcing" because it best described the sense that therapist/facilitators get through their hands as they tune in to the energy of energy cysts or any other active lesion.

It is as if the energy cysts are at the center point of an infinite number of concentric globes that are vibrating rotationally. Any specific point on the surface of any of the globes represents a small arc that is like the free end of a pendulum swinging to and fro, with the pendulum's central attachment at the center of the globe. The pendulum swing ignores gravity. In an arcing evaluation, each of the therapist/facilitator's hands usually perceives a slightly different arc, because the distance from the energy cyst is almost always different for each hand. Occasionally the central focus is equidistant from each hand. This can get confusing; the hands need to be moved to different positions to end the confusion. The problem lies in trying to project from each hand where the common central attachment for the two pendula is located, or where the projected radii of the two arcs would meet. These globes can be felt on or off the body. The number of globes is infinite. Therefore it doesn't matter what distance the

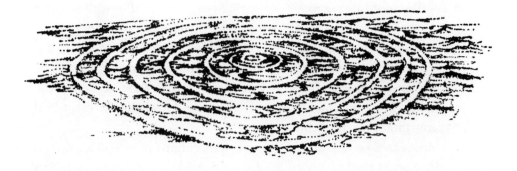

Illustration 2-1.
The concentric circles represent the waves of interference created by a pebble
dropped in the center of a pond. See text.

hands are from the energy cysts; they will feel the arcing activity.

The energy waves given off by the energy cyst might be considered analogous to the concentric ripples or interference waves given off when you drop a pebble onto the smooth surface of a pond. The natural, smooth wave activity of the pond might be likened to the craniosacral rhythm. The waves of interference superimposed on the pond surface by the disruption of the pebble might be seen as the phenomenon we are calling arcing.

In my experience, the rate of the rotational, rhythmical vibration of the waves emanating from the energy cyst is consistently more rapid than the rate of the craniosacral rhythm and slower than the heart rate. It seems not to be affected by the client's breathing.

The arcing system for energy cyst discovery and location has not changed appreciably since Dr. Karni and I developed it in 1976. Therapist/facilitators can place their hands anywhere on the body and use arcing to perceive the presence of an energy cyst anywhere else in the body—providing the effect is not diminished too greatly by distance or by the density of the medium through which the energy must travel.

As therapist/facilitators place their hands in different positions on and off the client's body, they can begin to zero in on the energy cyst by finding hand positions that locate arcs with smaller and smaller radii. When they are directly over the central focus (the energy cyst) for all the arcs, the sensation is like being above a pinwheel that rotates a short distance in one direction and then in the other. The rate of vibration is variable from one energy cyst to the next within the parameters of the heart rate at the high end and the craniosacral rhythm rate at the low end.

Palpation of obstructed acupuncture meridians may also lead to an energy cyst as the cause of the obstruction. An obstructed meridian could also be the residue of a previous problem that is no longer active. When I feel an empty or very full meridian, I take the time to manually trace that meridian along its course to discover whether an energy cyst is present. If there is one, there will also be arcing activity as I approach it, and I may well feel heat and other sensations.

I often find it interesting to practice Chinese pulse diagnosis to first locate a meridian problem by the pulses. I then palpate the meridian in its entirety (or as far as possible) in search of energy cyst blockage. If I find it, I correct it as I monitor the pulse. As the energy cyst is released, the Chinese pulse will change toward normal. If it is physically impossible to monitor pulses while releasing the energy cyst, the second best option is to recheck the pulse after energy cyst release is completed. This misses the process, but at least I can feel the effect of my treatment upon another body system.

Since our original work, my clinical observations have repeatedly shown that the energy cyst can cause pain, but it also can contribute to the formation of facilitated segments. In this way it may actually contribute to specific visceral disease in the future. The number of internal organ problems that can be caused either by energy cysts directly or by energy cyst contribution to segmental facilitation is inestimable.

I have also seen energy cysts with significant placement cause energy center/chakra dysfunction. I have had patients who spent years working on one or another energy center only to have it become dysfunctional soon after it was corrected. These patients may begin to

The Chakras

The seven "chakras," or wheels of energy, have been conceptualized by yogis in India since ancient times as centers of the ethereal body (energy body that engulfs the physical body). They take in vitality (prana) from the surrounding atmosphere; they are located along the central axis of the body; and they govern seven levels of the spiritual life of the yogic practitioner. The yogi strives to "awaken" or become conscious of these centers of energy through visualization and breathing exercises that concentrate attention on the areas in the body where they are located. These centers do not reside in the dimension of the physical body as such, though they are associated with major ganglia and organs of the physical body; rather, they reside in a subtle body that permeates and includes the gross physical matter. Each is in fact associated with a specific aspect of physical functioning and appears to be the center and energetic source of specific emotional qualities.

The root chakram is related to earth grounding. It is also said to be the seat of the "Kundalini" or fiery serpent. Kundalini is thought to be an energy derived from the sun, stored at the base of the spine. When liberated, it is thought to rush up the spinal cord to the brain, activating all the chakras as it passes through them. I have treated a few advanced yogis who said that CranioSacral Therapy enhanced and made easier the ascent of their Kundalini. The second chakram, sometimes called the "navel" or "power" chakram, is related to sexuality and power. It is often dysfunctional in those who have an unsatisfactory sexual life, especially those who trade sex for material support with no feelings of love. Opening this chakram and the heart chakram simultaneously will frequently improve and integrate sexual and love relationships. This chakram is also related to sensitivity, feelings and emotions, as well as the function of the liver, kidneys, intestines, and digestive organs.

The spleen or solar plexus chakram is related to the assimilation of energy and its distribution to other parts of the body; it is similar to the concept found in the acupuncture theory of the spleen as a refiner and distributor of chi to the other organs. Improving the function of this chakram will often improve immunity, resistance, and general activity levels. $\longrightarrow$

The heart chakram is frequently dysfunctional in those who have been hurt as children by someone in whom they had great trust. Now they are afraid to love for fear of being hurt again.

The throat chakram has to do with communication with other people and the ability to verbally express feelings.

The brow chakram is related to: a) the pituitary and pineal glands; b) clairvoyance and the ability to perceive things in connection with interpersonal relationships; and c) sensing the character of other persons and the purity of their motives.

The crown chakram is also related to the pineal gland and is the chakram that functions to establish a person's spiritual or cosmic connection.

Adapted from *CranioSacral Therapy II: Beyond the Dura, Glossary of Terms and Concepts*

blame themselves for having a spiritual defect that prevents them from achieving good and lasting chakra function. Often this self-blame is unwarranted, and the problem is corrected by release of an energy cyst.

I have not yet found a more effective method for the treatment of the energy cyst than to follow the body to its individual preferred position of release, the therapeutic position. The patient's body always seems to know best what it should do. A problem or obstacle to treatment may be presented by a part of the person that wishes to maintain status quo. The therapist/facilitator must identify the part of the client that wants to be relieved of the energy cyst and support it without offending the part that wants the status quo; both are trying to do the best they can for the person.

This kind of conflict within clients as it relates to an energy cyst usually shows itself as rapid, repetitive body movement that takes them to the edge of the therapeutic position and then speeds past it. When this kind of rapid movement occurs, I generally follow it for a few cycles to become familiar with the movement pattern. Then I slow it down. I become a slight inhibitory factor. I don't stop the movement, I just make the body part in question work a little to move my hands along with it. When I get to the edge of the therapeutic position, the craniosacral rhythm will stop suddenly. When this sudden stop occurs, I don't let the body part move past it; I hold it there. It usually feels as though it drops into a "notch." I now have the therapeutic position.

In my mind I characterize these rapid, repetitive movements as a manifestation of the internal debate within the patient. One part is saying, "Let's get rid of this nuisance, this energy cyst." The opposing part is saying, "Let's leave well enough alone. Why stir things up?" As the therapeutic facilitator, I am aligning my energy with the former of these two parts, saying, "If you want to get rid of this nuisance, I'll help you right now."

Sometimes, when it seems as though I am almost, but not quite, at the therapeutic position, the patient's nonconscious will actually test my dedication and skill. Dedication testing is carried out to see if the therapist/facilitator is patient and dedicated enough to go on the apparent wild goose chase necessary to get to the meat of the matter and stay with it. Skill testing is also carried out to see if the therapist/facilitator has the know-how to deal with the problem and its further developments once the energy cyst is dislodged and the release of its contents begins. In short, the client's nonconscious is testing the therapist's intention and skill.

Initiating the SER Process

The longer I practice as a therapeutic facilitator, the more I realize the power of intention. The kind of intention I use most often is an intention to support whatever the patient's "inner wisdom" wants to do at that time. My first intention, therefore, is to let the patient know that whatever he or she wants to do is okay with me. This is transmitted non-verbally through my initial touch. We will talk about many things. Our voices may be saying one thing and our touch communicating something entirely different. As the integration within the patient between conscious and nonconscious awareness progresses, we may very gently and with great sensitivity begin to verbalize what our touch communication has been considering since we began the session.

In practical terms this means that, when I first put my hands on a client, I silently say, "If you want to do CranioSacral Therapy that's what we'll do; show me where to begin. If you have a pressing issue with an energy cyst, that's okay; we'll do that. Show me where you would like me to be. If SomatoEmotional Release is what you want to do, just start and I'll be with you. Go ahead and image all you want. Please share those images with me. Perhaps I can help you understand what they are trying to tell you. We'll dialogue anytime you want to. Just let me know when you are ready. Whatever you think is the best way to come toward resolution of this problem is okay with me. Let's do it."

It is wonderful to see how the patient's body then begins to respond to this offering of help. I don't have to say a word until his body tells me to start talking. Small talk is a wonderful distracter, however; it helps the body get past the mind's defenses.

According to my best memory, the mystery of what I now call "intentioned touch" and "blending" came into my conscious awareness as early as 1954. It was shortly after I had finished my training as a hospital corpsman in the U.S. Coast Guard. I was placed on independent duty on a patrol ship in the Gulf of Mexico. Independent duty means that there are no other medically trained personnel aboard the ship. I had sixteen weeks of training and two months of internship in an outpatient clinic in New Orleans before being assigned to sea duty.

I was only on the ship a couple of days when the captain's steward sent word for me to see him. He was unable to walk due to a sudden pain in his left calf. He was lying on the deck grimacing and holding his leg as he writhed about. I was trained in life-saving procedures and really had no idea what to do. There were about six or seven crew members present; I felt them watching and judging my ability. The pressure was on—I could make it or break it right then.

I tried to look knowledgeable as I took his left leg between my two hands. I could feel a lot of heat and muscle contraction in his calf. I had no idea what the problem was, nor what I could do about it. I made my hands as gentle as I could and envisioned everything relaxing, the pain leaving, and all the blood vessels and nerves normalizing. Within two or three minutes the captain's steward smiled, said it felt fine, and thanked me. Then he stood up, tested his leg, continued to smile, and walked away. The onlookers smiled their approval and from that time forward started calling me "Doc."

I learned right then that if you intend to help the healing process and blend with the body tissues you are touching or holding, things will usually get better. By "blending" I mean that you consciously envision the boundaries between your hands and the other person's body dissolving and your hands entering the body. To better imagine how this might work, consider what happens when you have two bars of soap, one blue and one pink, and you place one atop the other, wet them, and wait. The two bars of soap merge at their areas of contact and the colors blend into each other. You may even see a lavender color as the blue and pink mix. Similarly, the energies of our bodies mix and integrate when we consciously intend it to happen. When the relatively normal energy of the therapist blends with the problem, it dilutes the problem energy and moves it towards normal. At the same time, if the therapist allows the problem energy to enter his or her body, an awareness of the problem can be perceived by the therapist. Since the entry of the problem into the therapist's body is consciously allowed by him or her, it can also be consciously removed by intention.

Today, my practice is to use intentioned touch to initiate SER. I touch the patient with silent statements about my intention. His or her body transmits my touch message to the nonconscious or higher intelligence, higher self, or whatever you prefer to call it. The touch, if sincerely well-intentioned and non-threatening, establishes a bond of trust between me and the patient's nonconscious (perhaps the conscious too, but I'm not as concerned with conscious awareness at the beginning). Once I establish trust, I may be tested a time or two. Sometimes I believe wild goose chases are activated to see if I really am willing to follow. Sometimes confrontations erupt to test my ego's stake in the process. And sometimes I get mixed messages that perhaps are sent to test my ability to follow patiently and adapt, or that represent conflict within the patient. I may be asked in many ways to prove my willingness to subordinate my ego. If I fail the test, all is not lost, however. It simply sets the process back a little—or perhaps all the way back to square one.

If, after I establish trust, a standing or sitting position for Somato-Emotional Release is desirable, I sense this information coming in through my hands. The patient's body will very subtly begin to move into a position. At this point it is important that I do not disbelieve what I am picking up. If the craniosacral rhythm stops and the patient's body seems to want to stand on its head, I go with it. I trust what my hands tell me. If I see an end position in my mind's eye, it is probably correct. Nonetheless, I wait for the patient's body to move to it on its own. Nothing is too weird, but I must wait for the patient to take me there—with a few exceptions. When I see an end position clearly and persistently, and the patient seems unable to get there, I may direct him to that place. The picture I am seeing probably is being put there by the patient's nonconscious, which may be saying I need to offer some leadership to get past the obstacles.

A good example of just such a situation came up during an Advanced CranioSacral Therapy class. I had to direct a person past a significant block to a strange place that challenged her ability to trust me. The subject in question was a fortyish woman therapist who had been repeating the same SomatoEmotional Release process over and over. I intervened to break the repetitive cycle and began to realize that she needed to re-enact her own birth process. Her repetitive cycle was apparently symbolic of her moving in space before she entered the fetus in her mother's uterus. Something was holding her back from entering the fetus that was already implanted. We helped her enter the fetus. Then her great fear of the delivery became apparent. There was also perceptible frustration with the way her obstetrical delivery had occurred. I began to see clearly that I would have to become the cervix located in her mother's body. The patient just couldn't get to it; she was really stuck. The image became more and more clear in my mind, so I finally decided to act on it. If the image was wrong, we would waste some time and have to start over; if the image was right, perhaps we could move past this "stuckness." I enacted what I saw in my mind's eye.

With the help of the rest of the therapeutic group, I put the patient on my shoulder and stood on the treatment table. I made a "cervix" with my hands. We held the patient head-down with her pelvis on my shoulder and her feet and legs up toward the ceiling. I really concentrated on being that cervix. The crown of her head pushed through the ring I formed with my thumbs and index fingers. As her head was "delivered" through my hands, I—the cervix—had to dilate more. Now I formed the cervical ring with my arms. First her shoulder began to pass through, then came her arm, then the other shoulder and the other arm. I maintained my arms as the cervical part of the birth canal; the four participating assistants supported her body from above and guided her down through my arms until her whole body was delivered and we were holding her in the air suspended by her ankles. The process took well over fifteen minutes. We had to go slowly and painstakingly; we had to be sensitive to every detail. It was very hard, physical work. We did not want to have to repeat it because we had overlooked some detail due to our fatigue or impatience.

Her "guides" seemed to be with us. [See chapter six.] We apparently followed the process correctly as it was laid out before us. The subject was very different after we completed the session. Today she is much happier and freer. She sent me a Mother's Day card thanking me for being a good cervix!

In this case I had to decide where to intervene upon a blocked repetitive process. I had to trust intuition even when it carried me into the ridiculously sublime transition of being a maternal cervix.

When therapists keep getting an image or impression, there may come a time when it is necessary to take the situation in hand and act upon that image to get past an obstacle. When they do this they have to be sure to recognize that they are leading. They have to be sure that they have left their personal psychological baggage out of the treatment session and that what they are going to act upon belongs to the client and not to them or someone else in the room. They have to proceed with their direction but always be willing to recognize that if it begins to feel wrong, the direction may in fact be inappropriate. Yet therapists can't be afraid to follow an incorrect process to a reasonable end point. They can't just stop and say something insensitive like, "Aw merde, this is wrong; we have to start over." I try to be soft and say something like, "Well, that was part of it. Let's go back and see if we have missed anything."

Multiple Facilitator SER

I used to believe that a competent individual therapeutic facilitator could do SER as well as a group of therapeutic facilitators; it would just take longer to get to the end result. I did concede that in a few instances, such as the example in which I was the maternal cervical canal, it might be impossible to physically re-enact an experience without extra muscle power from assistant therapeutic facilitators or just sensitive helpers who are willing to follow directions.

In retrospect, I believe I was trying very hard to keep SER within the practical grasp of those solo practitioners who wish to study and use this method. I continue to be convinced that most SER cases can be done by the unassisted, ego-subordinated, skilled therapeutic facilitator. It simply takes more time, greater patience, and requires the improvisational ingenuity that comes largely with time and experience in SER work. Still, it has been shown to me in the Advanced CranioSacral Therapy classes and in other contexts that there are times when the depth of release cannot be achieved as well by a solo therapeutic facilitator as it can be by a well-coordinated group providing extra energy, extra hands, and extra brains. In the Advanced CranioSacral Therapy class we are focusing more and more on developing a person's skill as an assistant therapeutic facilitator.

The assistant becomes an extension of the facilitator who is conducting the session with the client's nonconscious. The assistant is definitely part of the loop. He or she becomes an auxiliary perceptual station for the conductor, providing fresh perceptions and sensations. The assistant also blends with the client to better perceive and transmit information to the conductor. Insights that come to the assistant are shared with the conductor. The assistant should not act upon them without being instructed to do so. This relationship between conductor and assistants significantly enhances the therapeutic facilitator's energy, perceptual ability, intuitive insight, and intellectual potential. The level of enhancement depends upon the conductor's skill and sensitivity.

Where there is an experienced group of therapeutic facilitators working in harmony under the direction of an open conductor, the depth of penetration and degree of blending with a client is greatly increased. I do not believe that this depth of work can always be attained by a solo therapeutic facilitator, even over a protracted period. I have therefore revised my original stance on this issue. I encourage people training to become facilitators to spend perhaps one afternoon or evening per week working group-style with more difficult clients.

Completion of Biological Process: Birth, Death and Other Transitions

As time has passed and experiences have been gained, a most fascinating concept has been formulating. It seems that in SomatoEmotional Release we are repeatedly asked to "complete" obstetrical delivery processes from both the infant's and the mother's point of view. It is also very common to find the SomatoEmotional Release process completing a death transition or other transition process.

Perhaps I use the word "complete" incorrectly. The processes of delivery and transition to which I refer have been completed in an ordinary way. They seem not to have been completed, however, as judged from the point of view of some bioinstinct, morphogenetic energy field, gene, chromosome, DNA, or whatever. A naturally planned or predetermined process has somehow been thwarted.

I first began to clearly see this occur with patients who were delivered by Caesarean section. There is a significantly large number of craniosacral system dysfunctions in these patients that, unless corrected, will persist throughout life. I attribute this to the sudden change in fluid pressure that occurs when the uterus of a woman whose water has not been broken is quickly incised. This is, in fact, the case in many Caesarean-section deliveries. The baby is subject to a rapid decompression from higher intrauterine fluid pressure to lower extrauterine pressure. And make no mistake, this is a very rapid pressure change. I have seen amniotic fluid squirt out of a uterine incision as much as four inches into the air. This is analogous to a diver coming to the water's surface very rapidly from a significant depth. In infants it seems reasonable that the delicate membranes that are an intricate part of the craniosacral system may be strained or even slightly torn by this sudden pressure change. Adaptation to rapid decompression is a lot to ask of an infant. It is a tribute to the infant's resilience that more damage is not done. In any case, this explains the frequency of craniosacral dysfunction in people who are born by Caesarean section. But there is a further explanation.

Caesarean-section babies, in addition to being rapidly decompressed, miss their first natural "total-body treatment." This has been shown to me by patients who re-experience vaginal delivery via SomatoEmotional Release. As they twist their way through the process, cranial vault, cervical, thoracic, lumbar and pelvic releases occur. Pain sources become apparent and then often disappear. As the head passes through the birth canal, the bones overlap and the cranial vault slowly expands as the head presents itself. In normal birth, this is all done in good time, if the doctor or midwife is not too eager to get the process over.

All this became extremely clear to me when, in an Advanced CranioSacral Therapy class, I reprocessed my own vaginal delivery.

I shall never forget my sense of how the doctor wanted to pull me out. He pulled whenever he had a chance to get a finger hold on my head, mouth or chin. It was clear to me that I wanted to be born, but I wanted to go slowly, especially in certain phases of the process, because I could feel my body being correctly adjusted by the birth canal pressures, angulations, movements, and so on. I screamed silently to this well-meaning doctor, "Please leave me right here until this is finished. Then let me be pushed out as it was meant to be, not pulled out as you think it ought to be." During my session I was able, with the help of my own therapeutic facilitator, to modify this part of my delivery to serve my personal needs and desires. The modification has really helped my body.

The Caesarean-section infant is cheated out of the passage through the birth canal. I now view this passage as a very important part of the preparation for extrauterine life. Now, I thought, I surely had the total answer to the increased incidence of craniosacral system dysfunctions in Caesarean-section children. Wrong again, Upledger.

It has since been shown to me that a programmed process is put in place for both mother and fetus when the pregnancy begins. The fetus is supposed to go through its intrauterine development. We don't know whether this programming is directed by instinct, genetic patterning, the work of energy fields, or something that we don't yet understand. If the fetus does go through this development to the end, it will be pushed out of the uterus through a specially designed birth canal on a therapeutic trip in preparation for extrauterine life. When something such as a Caesarean section or forceps delivery interrupts or distorts this naturally intended process, there seems to occur some sort of retained biological frustration that can manifest in a variety of ways—most of which have to do with quality of function or chronic pain. When, during the SomatoEmotional Release process, the obstetrical delivery is completed as nature intended, the sense of biological frustration over the incompleteness of the process disappears, and the general functioning of the client significantly improves: pains disappear, obsessive compulsive behaviors lose potency, and so on.

What is true for the infant is true for the mother. When a pregnancy begins, it is as though a computer program is put into motion. This process is complete only when the birth is by vaginal delivery and mother-child bonding has occurred. When the natural process is thwarted, the biological process is incomplete. Again, incompleteness can manifest in many ways: Sometimes the woman is unable to conceive again; or there are various endocrine, nervous, behavioral, and pain problems. Once SomatoEmotional Release completes the biological program, many of these dysfunctions and symptoms correct themselves automatically.

The interruption of the birth process can occur in other ways besides Caesarean section and the rushing of delivery by impatient medical personnel. Many women today who are committed to their professional careers choose birth control to avoid pregnancy, or abortion when pregnancy occurs. As these women approach middle age, many become extremely anxious about not having given birth to a child. Because of their lifestyles, however, they still do not feel able to do so. In my view, there are biological reasons for their stress. I believe that the first menstrual cycle with ovulation may trigger a process that is not complete until pregnancy, delivery and maternal bonding have occurred. If the process is thwarted for any reason, it may cause the woman to desire to have a child "before it is too late."

In recent years we have been able to use SER to help such women resolve their conflict by undergoing pregnancy, birth and bonding on an imaginary level. It turns out that the biological process can be satisfied this way without an actual pregnancy.

I worked with five women over a period of two months with problems of this sort. Their biological clocks were ticking. They were all between thirty-five and forty years of age and had no children. They were all professionals enjoying various careers, and they were all experiencing similar inner conflicts about having a child before it was too late. There was a certain desperation about the situation for all of them. When this desperation gained the upper hand, each of them was tempted to go to a sperm bank, marry the first man who said yes to their proposal, or simply become pregnant by almost any man who would be a knowing or unknowing sperm donor.

These women were concerned about making at least a partial sacrifice of their careers to motherhood. The drive to be a mother is a very powerful one. I asked the first woman's Inner Physician if there might be an effective method of calming the drive without delivering a baby. The suggestion came to guide her through an imaginary pregnancy and delivery. I helped make this process as comfortable as possible by minimizing labor pains, suggesting that forceps were not necessary, and so on. When the baby was born the woman immediately bonded with her child's image! She nursed it, stayed with it, and loved it for several minutes; then, when she was ready, she let the baby go off into the cosmos. She felt it was a spiritual birth, and she released the spirit of the child when it was completed. Her Inner Physician approved of the process.

I kept in touch with this woman for a few months. Her strong drive to have a child seemed satisfied by imaging the whole process. She continued in her career and was no longer desperate or even concerned about entering the ranks of motherhood.

As fate seems to plan things, I soon had four more women much like this first one come to me for help. All four went through similar processes with me as their guide. And all four continued their careers without feeling driven to become mothers any longer.

The birth process is not the only process that is programmed by nature to pass through definite steps. It seems that the process of dying is also programmed. I say this first because of the many Somato-Emotional Release experiences where the client seems to regress to a previous lifetime for the purpose of re-experiencing his or her dying in a more acceptable way. Many facilitators of SomatoEmotional Release report being with clients who experienced or fantasized a past life and felt frustration with how it ended. Such people carry symptoms with them into this life that are related to that unsatisfactory death. These symptoms disappear spontaneously once the frustration, anger, guilt or fear from the past life or death in question is resolved. I used to think that the only significant goal for therapy was to resolve the destructive emotion attending such deaths. Now I'm thinking a little differently. It is as though the death process of the past life were incomplete. The resolution of destructive emotion also requires a qualitatively correct completion of the dying process.

Death is part of life, and nature says it must be completed properly. Perhaps part of that completion process is to review what we have done with our lives. Take stock of them. Evaluate what we have been shown. See what we have learned. Accept death as the end of another chapter in our existence. Once this is done, there seems no need to carry the sense of incompleteness with us any longer.

Another reason I say that the process is preprogrammed stems from my experience in the here and now with certain people as they linger before death. They seem stuck. Everyone can see that they are dying, but they seem to be taking too long to do it, showing much resistance, pain and suffering. Once a resolution of whatever incomplete life issue is reached, they are able to die. I'm sure if they die before they are ready, they will carry the biological incompleteness with them into a next life or into eternity. This incompleteness may serve to frustrate them until their previous life is brought to a proper completion.

My lesson in this began one night during my internship of 1963–64. I came onto the night shift and was confronted with a patient who had just returned from abdominal surgery. He was a man in his mid-forties who had come from Poland. He had cancer of the pancreas that had spread throughout his abdomen. The surgery had been an exploratory procedure. When the surgeons saw all the cancer growth, they decided to just close him up. They were unable to stop all the internal bleeding.

Before the surgery neither the man nor his family had any idea he was going to die. I came on duty to find this man just returned from the recovery room. I was told to keep him alive as long as I could, to notify his wife and family who were not at the hospital, and to obtain the last rites from a priest. The patient had two units of whole blood running, one into each of his arms. He also had IVs running into each of his legs.

I got acquainted with him both personally and physiologically. It was obvious that he could die at any moment. As I watched, his blood pressure dropped and he lost consciousness. I put some Aramine (a vasopressor to raise his blood pressure) through his IV tubing and he regained consciousness. He smiled and said, "I almost died, didn't I?"

I didn't want to say yes, but I did. How could I lie to this man? He asked me whether he could get better. I told him he was riddled with cancer and was bleeding inside. I told him I didn't see how he could get better, but that I would be with him all night and would do my best to do what he wanted.

He wanted to say good-bye to his wife who was at home, and he wanted the last rites from a Catholic priest. He went unconscious again as his blood pressure took another dive. I gave him another dose of Aramine. He came back, smiled and said, "Good work." I had never been so complimented in my life.

I quickly called his home. His brother answered the phone. I told him what was going on. He said he would be at the hospital within an hour with the wife, who didn't speak English.

The nurse called me back into the room. He was unconscious again and his blood pressure was way down. Aramine had worked twice, so I thought I would try it a third time. It did work, and he came back. I'll never forget how he looked me in the eye and said, "I almost died that time." I told him that his wife and brother were on their way, and that I was going to try to get a priest. I asked him to please hang on until we got all this stuff done. By now it was after 11 P.M. It was winter in Detroit and there was a blizzard outside. I called three parishes before I found a priest who said he would come in and give this man his last rites.

I went back in the room to find him fading again. More Aramine. The priest arrived before the wife and brother. He gave last rites, and I could see relief on the patient's face. The priest was just leaving when the wife and brother arrived. I gave the patient a little more Aramine so that he could talk to his wife and brother. I left the room. In a few minutes the brother came out and asked what I could do; his brother was unconscious. I went into the room with the idea that I would let him die this time.

His wife looked pleadingly into my eyes. I gave him more Aramine. He came back again and said, "Thank you. I want a little more time, if you can do it, to make my wife feel better." Feeling as though I was in Rod Serling's other dimension, I left the room totally confused about my values and the position I found myself in. His wife came out shortly and gave me that look again. I went in and gave him more Aramine. He came back, but this time he said, "I can go now, you don't need to bring me back anymore." He left about forty-five minutes later for the last time.

I thought about that experience for quite awhile. He knew when he had brought his process to completion. He had not been forewarned that this was to be the last night of this incarnate life. It took him a few hours to get it all in order, reach a resolution, and allow the process to go to completion. I'm sure that had he died before receiving the last rites or before talking with his brother and his wife, he would have died prematurely. Even though it was a question of only a couple of hours, the process would perhaps have been thwarted if he had died prematurely. He would have died frustrated and angry—and perhaps carried these destructive feelings into his next life. Part of our work as therapeutic facilitators is to help prepare the client for a nice, clean entry into the next life. I really believe those few hours of meaningfully extended life made a great deal of difference to him.

Sometimes there may be a physiological reason for the "stuckness" that interferes with the death process. An osteopath with whom I am very close sent me a letter about an experience she had that said it all. She had a patient in the hospital who was dying of lung cancer. She was dying in great distress and with great effort. My friend simply touched the patient's cranial vault. The vault was in marked extension and was stuck there. My friend then exaggerated the extension and a release occurred. The cranial vault went into a large flexion cycle. The patient smiled, took one very deep, relaxed breath, and died with a smile on her face. Perhaps her physiological dying process got stuck.

Some New Experiences

During 1989, two very significant lessons were presented to me. I'll share them and you can make of them what you wish. Both incidents occurred while I was working in our Brain and Spinal Cord Dysfunction Center with patients who were there for our two-week intensive program.

The first involved a male patient in his thirties. He had been one of the victims of a Los Angeles freeway sniper. The bullet had entered behind his left ear, passed through his skull, and lodged in the back of his neck, partially shattering two vertebrae. The patient couldn't talk and was in a wheelchair. We were having a lot of trouble extracting an energy cyst from his head and neck. It then occurred to me that we had to connect with the anger or insanity of the shooter to release the energy cyst.

I simply asked the shooter's emotional energy to come out of the wound. I made this request aloud. There were several of us working during this session. We all felt the rage and insanity as the energy cyst slowly released from behind the left ear. Over and over in my mind I kept hearing the shooter screaming, "F____ you! F____ you!"

This patient got off his plateau after this session. His attitude improved, he showed signs of talking, and he regained a little motor control and sensation in his legs.

The second experience was with two teenage girls who were riding in the same car when it was hit by another car. Both had amnesia about much of the accident. Following our intuition, we put the two patients on parallel tables. I positioned myself between them with the driver on my left and the passenger on my right.

We were able to re-experience the accident together and release the forces that went into the car in which they had been riding. As we did so, much anger that had previously been denied surfaced, and we talked about the driver of the other car. One of these patients was wheelchair-bound and the other had some third and fifth cranial-nerve deficit that was residual. It was a most effective session. We actually elicited a little sympathy for how the driver of the other car must feel. We had previously worked intensively on both patients and had been unable to re-experience the accident, unable to connect with repressed anger, and certainly unable to get them to consider how the driver of the other car must feel about the damage that resulted from the accident.

The girl in the wheelchair can now support her full weight on her right leg as a result of the session described above. Both girls are now willing to meet and discuss the accident with the woman who hit them.

Chapter Three

Vector/Axis Integration and Alignment

The technique we have named "Vector/Axis Integration and Alignment" is something I have been doing intuitively and largely in a nonconscious way for more than twenty-five years. As a diagnostic and therapeutic tool, it works very well in conjunction with CranioSacral Therapy in facilitating SomatoEmotional Release.

During an Advanced CranioSacral Therapy seminar in the early 1980s, one of the students, named Adam, asked me what exactly I was doing. I evaded giving a precise answer. He repeated his question rather insistently. I realized that I was aware of neither what I was doing nor why.

Whatever it was, it happened as I allowed my hands and the rest of my body to do what felt appropriate for the patient. It was very subtle. It involved use of the extremities in movements of tractioning (pulling), torquing (twisting), side bending, compressing, waiting, and so on. Most of the passive movements I performed on the patient's body were very small. On occasion, however, I would move the ankles several inches to accomplish an effect in the torso. I always felt a sort of "falling into place" at the correct position. After this occurred there was a sense of stabilization or melding into position. This work was usually the finishing touch.

Adam continued his questioning and the rest of the group began to gather around. I was trying to formulate answers while standing at the supine patient's feet. Suddenly I "saw" sparkling, very active, energetic lines superimposed within, not on, the patient's body. Structurally they resembled the stick figures that most of us draw as children. The lines were so shiny and energetic that they looked like Fourth of July sparklers. In this first instance, the sparkling lines all appeared to be within the patient's body. (Since then, I frequently have seen them on the outside of patients.)

There was one line from the lower abdomen straight up the center of the body to the head, but it was interrupted just below the solar plexus. There were two horizontal sparkling lines. One ran from shoulder to shoulder and the other from hip to hip. These lines connected with the sparkling, interrupted, centrally located vertical line. At the lateral ends of both horizontal lines were "hinges" that allowed them to tilt relative to the arms and legs, and to extend in each arm from shoulder to hand and in each leg from hip to foot. The hinge at the right shoulder seemed somehow disrupted. The right arm line was not actually connected to the shoulder-to-shoulder line. The line through the hips was tilted about ten degrees. The right end was above and the left end was below, but the hinges were connected so that the sparkling lines in the legs were connected to the line through the hips. Although the sparkling lines would have been consistent with unequal physical leg length, the legs were of equal length.

I pointed out these sparkling lines to Adam and the rest of the group who had gathered around. Adam immediately asked what they were—he could see them too! Without hesitation I heard myself say that the lines were "vectors." (A vector is a line with a direction, like an arrow.) Vectors of what, I did not know. It did seem that these vectors were highly energetic. It also seemed that the disruptions at the level of the solar plexus and in the right shoulder hinge should somehow be connected, and that the vector from hip to hip should be repositioned from a diagonal position to one parallel to the ground.

As you might guess, the next question from the students was, "What do we do with those vectors?" I heard myself reply without hesitation that we would simply put them together where the continuity was disrupted and straighten, balance, or reposition as indicated. At

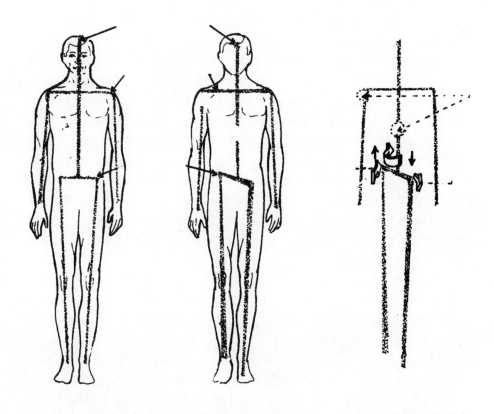

Illustration 3-1.
Comparison of ideal vector/axis system (left) with the system we visualized (middle).
On the right the vector/axis system has been extracted from the body for clarification.

this point, I realized that this was what I had been doing nonconsciously and intuitively for so many years.

To demonstrate to the class how I would go about integrating and
aligning this patient's "vector system," I had to allow my hands to
have their way. It was a moment of truth. Was I being permitted to
"see" what I had been working with all along, or were these two separate systems I sensed—one with my hands and one with my eyes?
Would the movements of my hands with the patient's body connect the
disruptions in the vector system that I was seeing for the first time?

I thought how fortunate it was that the Advanced class had only ten people. One of them was the patient on the table. We were all good friends by now, so I wouldn't be making a fool of myself in front of a large, possibly antagonistic audience if this didn't work as I intuited it would. I let my hands tell me what to do. We saw the vectors reconnect where they were disconnected. As a group we could kinesthetically sense when the separated ends came together, and we could feel when they were securely melded into a single vector. It was not as obvious kinesthetically when the diagonal hip-to-hip vector moved, but we could see it happening. When the position of balance was achieved, there was a sense of "falling into place." Most of the students felt this phenomenon occur. It was exciting to be able to "see" the effect of what I was doing. I shall now attempt to describe what I did.

First, I decided to balance the relationship of the horizontal pelvic hip-to-hip vector with the vertical central vector. This decision was arbitrarily intuitive. I am sure that I would have done just as well if I had integrated and aligned the right arm with the right shoulder. I did horizontal-vertical vector alignment by simply pulling on the right leg and simultaneously pushing in the left leg very gently. The focus of attention was at the hips, which I moved by using the legs as long levers. My hand contact with the patient's body was at the feet. I was cradling one heel in each hand. I was lifting the feet and legs to the upper thigh area, just slightly up and off the table to reduce body friction with the table top. As the vector appeared to align horizontally, I became aware that there was an abnormal rotation around a vertical axis. The right lateral end of the horizontal vector was in back and the left lateral end was in front.

I want to emphasize that none of these vector misalignments had any correlation to physical body misalignment. We can use the physical body, however, to move the vectors if we go slowly and carefully. It is as if a magnetic attraction exists between the physical body and the vector when the system is energized adequately.

I rotated the pelvis a little in a counterclockwise direction from my vantage point at the feet. I continued until the "falling into place"

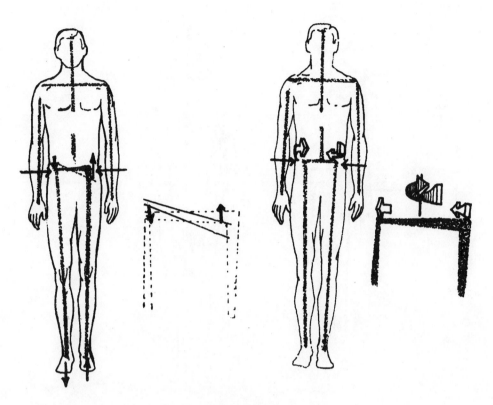

Illustration 3-2.
Shows how transverse hip-to-hip vector/axis was corrected in relationship
to the vertical central vector/axis. See text.

sensation was felt by me and the rest of the class, who were not touching the patient. Once I felt this "falling into place," it seemed proper to wait a few seconds (perhaps ten) until the vector appeared to settle in and be "happy" in its realigned position. I have found that if you move the body too soon after achieving the desired vector alignment, you can lose vector continuity, or the vector will distort again as you replace the body parts in question.

Next, I reattached the right arm vector to the shoulder. I straightened the arm until the arm vector was on a horizontal line with the shoulder vector. Then I pushed in the arm until I could see the two

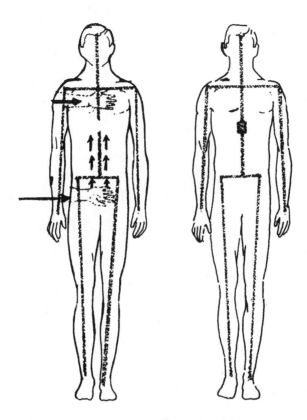

Illustration 3-3.
Method used to reconnect the infradiaphragmatic disruption
of the central vector/axis. See text.

ends of the disconnected vectors come together. At this point, kinesthetic sense and intuition took over. I felt the two ends come together.
They felt as though some sort of "hooking" was required, much as
you might hook or rotate the arm of a mannequin into position to
attach it. I rotated just about ninety degrees counterclockwise, as
though to line up the mechanism. I then slowly rotated about sixty
degrees clockwise until I felt the arm fall into place. The students
also felt this sensation. Again I waited, perhaps thirty seconds this
time, until the vector union seemed stable to me. This sensation of
stability was like a sigh of relief as the two vectors melded. Every-

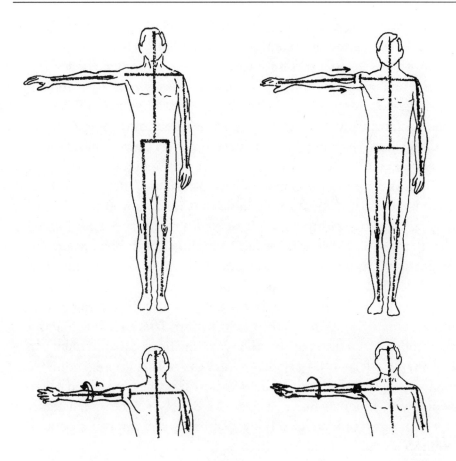

Illustration 3-4.
Shows steps used in reconnecting and aligning the vector/axis of the right arm
with the lateral end of the shoulder-to-shoulder transverse vector/axis. See text.

one in the room with me seemed to know when the melding was complete.

Next, I placed one hand under the sacrum and the other hand under the lower thoracic spinal region. I compressed the lower spine into the thoracic region until I could see and feel a connection of the disrupted area in the solar plexus vector. We all felt it when the ends touched. We waited for a few seconds until it seemed stable, then I took my hands away. Re-examination of the patient using the visualization of the shiny, sparkling lines revealed an integrated and highly energetic, visible vector system within his body.

I must confess that this initial attempt to comprehend, visualize, explain, and teach these little finishing touches was pretty astonishing to all of us. After this first demonstration we had two full days of class remaining. We continued to experiment and play with the sparkling lines, the concepts and the techniques. It was a mind-blowing two days. Here we were, all pretty much seeing the previously invisible and feeling the previously "non-feelable." In view of these circumstances, it is most remarkable that we achieved a high level of agreement regarding what we sensed. I'm not sure that I know what to make of this sudden piece of insight, or of the expansion and integration of my visual and kinesthetic abilities onto a conscious level. I do know that it is a teachable technique.

Since that first experience, I have put this subject into the format of the SomatoEmotional Release workshop. There we teach about sixty students at a time to "see" the sparkling lines. Most of them can do it in one afternoon. I also know that the results are reproducible and that everyone who experiences Vector/Axis Integration and Alignment is very much aware of its positive effects. Clients consistently express a sense of increased body awareness and improved general "connectedness."

I put in the word "axis" when naming this method because "vector" implies motion or force. This is not always the case. I do not wish to imply that a directed force is always a component of these sparkling lines. On the other hand, there does seem to be a direction of energetic force in some people. Therefore, for the sake of clarity, I have begun using the combined term vector/axis for the visualized sparkling lines that we see superimposed in the client. Many therapists see the lines with individualized characteristics. Some see them as blue lines, some as gold or yellow, and so on. I can only tell you how I see them.

One of the first people we tried our new technique on in a clinical situation was a male lead dancer from a major ballet company. He had been dancing with this ballet troupe for about six years when he was afflicted with a non-malignant tumor of the spinal cord. The tumor had been successfully excised about six months before I saw him. His recovery had been without incident or complication, and physical therapy had begun shortly after surgery, yet he was far from symptom-free.

At the time he came to our facility he was walking with a cane. His gait was stiff and tentative. He swung his legs laterally a bit as he walked. He stated that he was having a very difficult time making his legs do what he wanted them to do. As a dancer, he was used to having his body do just what he asked of it. He was also used to knowing, without using his eyes, exactly where his body parts were. He had lost some of this knowledge. His body performance and awareness expectations and requirements were naturally much greater than those of the average person.

He came to us for two weeks of treatment. He had a total of eight appointments with me. My first and dominant finding was a lack of longitudinal mobility of the dural tube. It was very restricted in the middle and lower thoracic region. I spent the first two and a half to three sessions almost completely focused on dural tube mobilization. I worked it from both ends using the occipital and sacral handles. Some of our time had to be invested in the mobilization of these handles. I used multiple CV-4 techniques to force fluid down the dural tube. I performed V-spread techniques from front to back through the thorax, as well as between the top of the head and the base of the spine in both top-to-bottom and bottom-to-top directions.

It takes some time to direct energy the total length of the dural tube, but it is well worth the investment. The V-spread technique involves sending energy from one hand toward the other and continuing to send it until you feel its arrival in the receiving hand. You have to take your time and make sure that you do it correctly and that you complete the task. When the task is done, you feel pulsation, heat and, finally, a sense of release in your receiving hand.

With the dural tube mobilized, the patient noticed an immediate

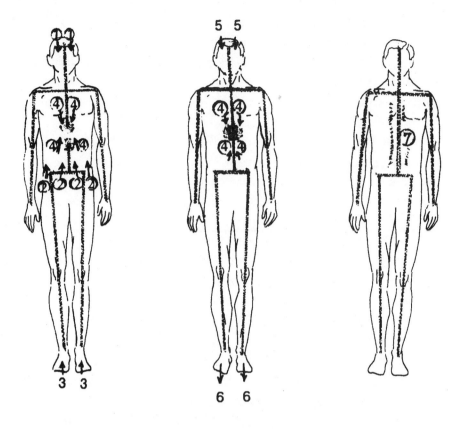

Illustration 3-5.
Shows the steps used in reconnecting the central vertical vector/axis after surgical excision of a spinal cord tumor. See text. 1) Compression of head into trunk in attempt to approximate disrupted vector/axis ends—unsuccessful. 2) Similar attempt at approximation from pelvis—unsuccessful. 3) Similar attempt at approximation from feet—unsuccessful. 4) Achieved approximation working locally at site of interruption of vector/axis continuity. 5) Compression of head into body is now helpful. 6) Traction at feet does not disconnect vertical vector/axis. 7) Integrity of vector is maintained.

improvement in motor coordination. His legs obeyed commands they had not obeyed for some time; his knees bent more readily and as he directed. By the end of the first week, his motor coordination was significantly improved in his opinion, but his internal awareness of body position had not improved as much as he wished. When he did a leap, he wasn't sure when his feet would touch the floor or whether they were in the correct position.

I tried Vector/Axis Integration and Alignment. This was about three weeks after my first experience with the sparkling lines. I saw a very prominent disruption of his central vertical vector/axis. The gap between the two disconnected ends was about six inches long. It ran from the middle of his chest into his belly. The task was to fill the gap in order to meld the two ends of the disconnected vector/axis. I tried pushing in energy from his head down, from his pelvis up, and finally from his feet upwards. As I watched I could see the sparkling energy building at the disconnected ends, but the ends did not get closer to each other. I decided to try to bring these ends together manually at the site of the disruption in the central vector/axis continuity.

This simplistic approach seemed a little off the wall at the time, even to me. But what was there to lose? I knew I couldn't hurt anything, so I tried. It took a couple of minutes before anything happened, then the disconnected ends began to move toward each other, closing the gap. In a short time they abutted each other, but the ends did not seem to meld together. I went back to the patient's head and gently pushed in a downward direction, holding this push until I felt the now familiar "falling into place" sensation. This sensation was followed by a sense that the two ends were melding together. Next there was a sense of relaxation, as though the resistance had gone. I then went to his feet and gently tractioned down. The central vertical vector/axis maintained its integrity. His vector/axis system seemed normal, intact, and very "sparkly" to me. I asked him to try it out. He did not ask me what I had done, and I did not volunteer any explanation.

The next day he reported that for the first time since his tumor began to bother him, he knew exactly where his feet were when he leaped into the air and returned to the floor. He knew precisely when they were about to strike the floor, and he felt in total control of the position of his feet and legs as he landed. We both rejoiced and were astonished at how quickly his body awareness had returned after this session of Vector/Axis Integration and Alignment. It was as though it had never been gone. I spent the rest of his sessions exercising his craniosacral system, increasing his dural tube mobility, and re-evaluating his vector/axis system. Actually, there was little left for me to do, but I kept looking for more even though I didn't find it. His craniosacral system and vector/axis system remained intact and in excellent working order.

Since that first emergence of the vector/axis system, I have received several reports from others to whom we presented this technique. The clinical results on a subjective and anecdotal level seem to be quite excellent. The techniques have been rapidly assimilated into several therapists' armamentarium. The beauty of the concept seems to echo the whole of CranioSacral Therapy: It is a no-risk technique; it consumes minimal time, but the time must be one-on-one with the patient; and it is an open-ended technique. Just as CranioSacral Therapy forces therapists to develop their perceptions, skills, attitudes and thinking so that new vistas open for them, so does Vector/Axis Integration and Alignment. For those who practice this technique, it develops and expands their sensory limits. An unknown universe awaits further exploration.

Now let us consider some further clinical observations I have made and that have been reported to me since we first added Vector/Axis Integration and Alignment to our curriculum. Sometimes the vectors/axes are outside the boundaries of the physical body. In such cases I use the physical body, much as I would a magnet, to collect the vector/axis that is displaced. After the vector/axis settles into the body and stabilizes itself, the body is used to manipulate the vector/axis into its correct position of alignment or to reconnect the separated end of a disrupted area.

One must allow time for the vector/axis to meld into the proper position in the physical body before attempting to use the body as a vehicle to move the vector/axis. It is as though the body can be used as a time-lapse magnet for the vector/axis. If the physical body is moved too soon or too fast, the vector/axis is lost. That is, the magnetic

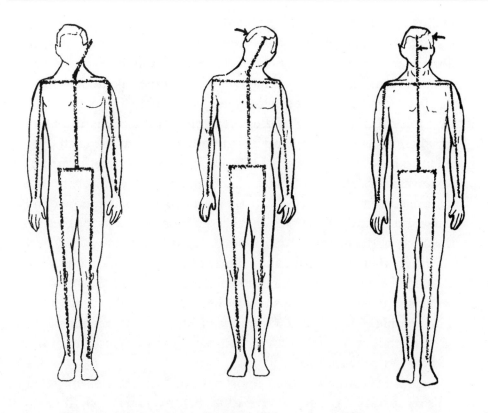

Illustration 3-6.
Shows use of the physical head and neck to "collect" an energetic vector/axis that is displaced from the physical body and return it to a normal position. See text.

attraction between the physical body and the vector/axis is overcome. If this happens, no harm is done. One can just go back, collect the vector/axis, and try again.

Vector/axis continuity is definitely disrupted or distorted by energy cysts, somatic dysfunctions, physical trauma, emotional disturbances, and the like. If one integrates and realigns the vector/axis system but does not resolve the underlying problem, the vector/axis will move back into its disrupted or misaligned pattern very quickly. I occasionally have seen this return to abnormality occur in a matter of seconds. This characteristic has an up side to it: The system can be used

to discover whether there is an underlying physical or emotional problem that has gone either undetected or unresolved and is causing the
disruption or misalignment of the vector/axis system.

With some ingenuity, therapists can determine a great deal about
the nature and significance of the underlying problem from the rapid-
ity, location and severity of the recurring vector/axis disruption or
misalignment. They can learn about body parts that the client considers to have committed offending acts or to not have performed up
to demand or expectation, and thus have been rejected. There may
be resistance to getting well. Or there may be missed energy cysts,
missed somatic dysfunctions, or other emotional reasons for the continuation of the repetitive disruption of the vector/axis system.

Once, when demonstrating before a SomatoEmotional Release
class, I did a successful reconnection of a separated central vertical vec-
tor/axis. This separation was below the waist. The subject was a student volunteer. Within a few seconds of finishing the reconnection,
several student observers and I witnessed the reseparation of this
central vertical vector/axis.

Again, I reconnected the vector/axis and it promptly separated.
This reseparation occurred three times before I caught on. After the
third reconnection and separation, the volunteer student went into
a SomatoEmotional Release process that involved re-experiencing
and releasing the effects of an unwanted pregnancy and abortion.
She then completed a natural obstetrical delivery process as though
the pregnancy had gone to completion. She also confronted and
resolved the hidden guilt about killing her baby through the abortion. She confronted and accepted her sexuality, though it was her
sex drive that had gotten her into this predicament initially. In essence,
she came face-to-face with her libido, the existence of which she had
tried to deny since her pregnancy and abortion.

In her attempt to deny her sexuality and the existence and character of her libido, she had interrupted the continuity of her vertical
central vector/axis between the waist and the pubic region. Before
we could get a lasting reconnection of this central vector/axis, she

had to forgive herself and accept her sexuality as being a natural part of who she was. With some dialogue and negotiation, she readmitted her pelvis and its organs to her total being. She forgave herself. The vector/axis was then reconnected and remained intact.

Since that experience, I have become aware of several cases of emotionally based body-part rejection that manifested as vector/axis separations and misalignments. A very interesting example is that of a young man whose complaint was of right arm and shoulder pain. He could think of no particular incident or injury that might have caused the pain. He just woke up with it one morning. He had received several types of treatment, but the problem did not respond to any of them. It seemed to be getting progressively worse. It was not really an acute problem, but it was enough to prevent him from throwing a baseball or passing a football with his son. The patient had been a quarterback on his high-school football team and wanted very much for his son, now twelve years old, to excel on the high-school team in a few years.

During the first visit we went through an energy cyst release that was mostly physical. After this session I noted that the right arm vector was disconnected from the lateral end of its transverse shoulder vector/axis. Also, the right side of the transverse shoulder vector/axis was disconnected from the central vertical vector/axis. I straightened the arm to horizontal and compressed medially, attempting to attach both separations simultaneously. I was successful. The reconnection lasted for three minutes, then it went right back to the double separation.

On the next visit, SomatoEmotional Release revealed that he was rejecting his right arm because of a bad pass he had thrown in an "important" football game. The pass was intercepted and the game was lost. This was his last game as a high-school football player. He did not attend college, so it was the end of his football career. He was really angry with his right arm and shoulder. They had performed badly at a very important time in his life. As his son's entry into high school loomed closer, and as he tried to teach his son to be a quarterback and pass a football, his rejected arm and shoulder became more and more symptomatic.

Through dialogue and negotiation with his arm and shoulder, an amicable relationship was achieved. He forgave and accepted his arm and shoulder. I reconnected the vector/axis system where it was separated (as in Illustration 3-7). This time the reconnection held. His arm and shoulder function returned to normal. (I hope his son doesn't take his football career as seriously as his father did!)

After a period of working with Vector/Axis Integration, I realized I had been using it intuitively with scoliosis (spinal curvature) patients for some time.

Before I get into the vector/axis system part, I should give you some background about how I view and treat scoliosis. First, I use arcing to search for specific active lesions along the torso. I look for the lesion that is key to the spinal curvature. My idea is that the small muscles between or along vertebrae that are strained could be sending incorrect information to the large muscles that are involved in maintaining postural stance. I search for these strained small muscles and attempt to relax them. I couple this approach with a balancing of the craniosacral system.

Once I accomplish this, I mobilize and balance the vertebral column, the pelvis and the extremities. I also investigate possible emotional reasons for spinal curvature. These emotional reasons, when present, may well cause recurrent distortions of the vertical central "sparkling line."

At this point I have already essentially removed, as best I can, all the factors that cause distortions and disruptions in the vector/axis system. At the end of each session I realign and integrate the vector/axis system. I use it as an index to reflect the ongoing presence of dysfunctions, energy cysts, and emotions that may continue to disrupt the system's organization and integrity.

Besides this use of the vector/axis system, I have a strong feeling that if we can maintain the straightness of the central vector/axis and achieve spinal mobility at the same time, the straightness of the central vector/axis will influence, albeit slowly, the mobile spine toward

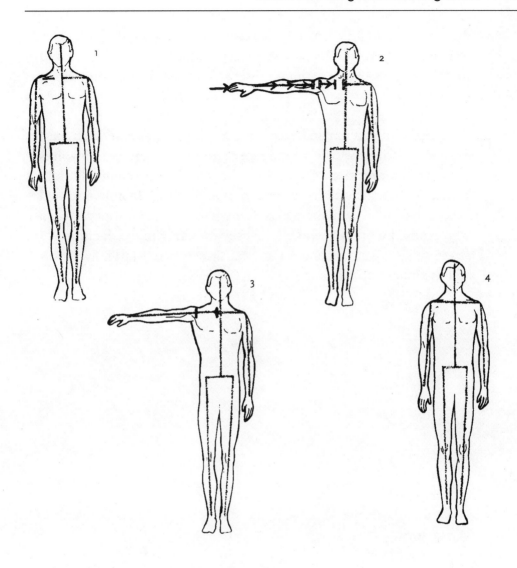

Illustration 3-7.
1) Interruptions in shoulder-to-shoulder horizontal vector/axis adjacent to central vector/axis and at right lateral end where it connects to the arm. 2) Position of reconnection. 3) Reconnection occurs. 4) Return to normal. See text.

straightness. It is therefore important that the scoliotic patient be seen once or twice a week, because keeping the central vector/axis as straight as possible for as much time as possible during the week is vital.

Vector/Axis Integration and Alignment has become an important part of my diagnostic and therapeutic repertoire. As you can see, it involves the skillful application of awareness, together with an equally skillful use of a very specialized form of imagination. In conventional approaches to medical diagnosis, imagination is strictly taboo, yet a therapeutic facilitator who suppresses the imaginative faculty will never see the "sparkling lines." I am learning every day just how important the imagination can be.

Chapter Four

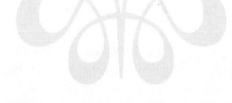

Therapeutic Imagery and Dialogue

The purpose of this chapter is to introduce the Inner Physician and other internal figures that arise in the course of therapy through the use of the imagination. The Inner Physician is a real and imaginary being who exists in every person and is usually perfectly well-informed about the health condition of that person, what the reasons are for his or her symptoms, and what can be done to alleviate the symptoms. What do I mean by real and imaginary? We will see ...

Imagination, Fantasy and Talking to Yourself

It is bedtime. The light in my room is off, but my bedroom door is ajar and some light from the hallway is coming in. Mom has tucked me in and kissed me goodnight. She doesn't understand about the monster in my closet. The monster always tries to get me when the light in my room is turned off and I'm supposed to sleep. He is looking out of the closet now and I can see his yellow eyes shining. He wants to kidnap me and take me away forever. He starts to come out of the closet. I'm so scared. My heart is pounding out of my chest and I can't make a sound.

Just in the nick of time, my angel Jennifer appears on the windowsill, all shiny and sparkly. All she has to do is point her magic wand at the monster and he stops in his tracks. Then he slowly starts to back into the closet where he stays. He looks at Jennifer and makes ugly faces at her.

Jennifer says, "John, don't be so afraid. I'll always be here to protect you." I still can't make a sound or move a muscle, but my heart quiets down a little. Jennifer comes closer and spreads some magic dust on me so that I can talk and move. Jennifer says again, "John, I really will protect you from the monster."

And I say, "But what if you don't get here in time and the monster takes me into the closet with him? He has a secret tunnel from the closet to Monsterland, and if he gets me there I'll never get back."

Jennifer replies, "John, please believe me. I really won't ever let the monster take you away or hurt you even a little bit."

"But Jennifer, what if he sneaks out of the closet when you aren't watching and takes me where you can never find me?"

"John," it's my mother's voice as she enters my bedroom, "are you talking about monsters again? And who are you talking to?" Mom turns on my bedroom light. "See, there isn't anyone here. Who are you talking to?"

I try to tell Mom about the monster in the closet who comes out to get me when the bedroom light is off. "But you're still here," Mom says. "The monster didn't get you." Opening the closet door and turning on the lights, she adds, "And look! There isn't any monster in the closet." I can't look, I'm afraid.

"And who were you talking to about the monsters?" Mom asks.

"I was talking to my angel, Jennifer. She saved me. She scared the monster away."

"That's enough foolishness. Go to sleep, it's late. Forget about monsters and angels. There isn't anyone here. You are letting your imagination run away with you. You've got to stop imagining things."

I feel humiliated and frustrated. Mom never believes me about the monsters or about Jennifer. Why won't she believe me?

For my fifth birthday, a dream came true. I got a 12-bass accordion and beginner's lessons at the Wurlitzer Music Studio in Detroit. When I was three, we had a New Year's Eve party at our house, and a man came over with his accordion—a "stomach squeezer" I called it. I was entranced. Dad bought me a little toy concertina to placate me until I was old enough to get a real accordion and lessons at Wurl-itzer. I was so excited. After a few lessons I started to learn some basic, familiar songs like "Jingle Bells" and "La Golendrina." In a very short time I was adding a few little creative licks of my own to these songs.

Each time I demonstrated my own creative improvisation, my teacher rapped the music stand with her baton. She told me to play the music just as it was written. Soon I began to stand up for myself, telling her it sounded better my way. She would then tell me that it would take some years before I could write my own music. Until then, I had to play it like it was written. The accordion lost a lot of its appeal when I had to do it strictly her way.

Fortunately, Dad saw the problem and wisely intervened. He began giving me a dollar each time I got a gold star for my lesson. I could buy three sheets of popular music with that! Once I had the sheet music with the words and the melody, I could sing and play the song any way I wanted to. Not many aspiring musicians have the kind of father who will nurture individual creativity in contradiction to the system. I was extremely fortunate.

I was in third grade. It was spring. Spring fever was upon me. My seat in the classroom was toward the back of the room near the window. All I could think about was the outdoors—how blue the sky was, how billowy and fluffy the clouds were, how warm the sun was. Why did I have to sit here in this classroom, able only to dream of the outdoors and freedom? Soon my attention was captured by a hawk making circles in the sky. I kept watching him as he glided gracefully through the sky. Suddenly I was in an open-cockpit biplane. I followed the hawk doing his circles.

In only a second or two I had become an aviator. I was flying my own airplane. As I followed the hawk, I got closer and closer. Finally I was flying beside him. I asked him what he was doing. He replied that he was practicing to be the world's best-flying hawk. I was truly impressed. I asked if he minded if I flew along with him.

He said, "Not at all," and suggested that, so long as we were going to fly together, I should call him by his first name, Henry. I told him my name was John. He said, "Hello, John. I'm pleased to meet you." My grandfather always said, "Likewise, I'm sure"; so I said, "Henry, it's likewise, I'm sure." Suddenly we were good friends.

I told Henry that if he was practicing to be the world's best-flying hawk and I did what he did follow-the-leader style, I could probably become the world's best aviator. Henry thought that made sense and agreed to lead me through the stunts he knew. Soon we were doing loop-the-loops, stalls, dives and figure eights, and I was right on his tail feathers.

As I became more involved in the follow-the-leader exercise, I must have put my arms out like airplane wings and made roaring biplane-engine noises, because just when I was getting really hot, I was brought down to earth by a firm grip and pull on my right ear by my teacher.

"Come back down to earth, young man. That's enough day-dreaming. We have work to do. If you don't get finished, you will have to go to summer school," she told me in a stern, no-nonsense voice. I learned right then that fantasy is not allowed in the third grade.

These experiences are similar to those that occur in many of our lives. They serve to demonstrate that fantasy, imagination, talking to yourself, and so on, are seriously discouraged from very early on at home and in most school systems. Because success in most schools depends largely on "paying attention," "being real," memorizing, and parroting, most parents try to get their children to let go of any embarrassing fantasy life at a fairly early age. Fantasy just isn't productive. There may even be something "wrong" with the child who over-indulges in fantasy.

I had occasion to work with and develop a rather deep friendship with a world-renowned psychic who had stayed in the closet about her talents until she was about forty years old. Why? Because during the flu epidemic of 1918, when she was a very little girl, she went around the neighborhood wearing a little nurse's hat and putting her hands on flu victims' foreheads. Those people she touched got better. They told her mother about it. Her mother spanked her and told her not to do that anymore; it was bad. She said it wasn't normal to be able to do that, and only witches did those kinds of things.

Therapeutic facilitators who make use of therapeutic imagery and dialogue in their work have this kind of negative indoctrination to overcome in many of their clients. Yet what is therapeutic imagery but active imagination, and this kind of dialogue but talking to yourself? Usually if you talk to yourself enough you get to spend some time in a rubber room; you might even get some drugs to inhibit your creative images and stop you from talking to them if they do form. So imagine being a therapeutic facilitator trying to convince the client's brow-beaten, insulted and inhibited creative energies that it is safe to come out and show themselves and everyone else what they can do.

The fact that these creative talents are present in most of us is demonstrated by the wonderful success of Bill Cosby, Whoopi Goldberg, Robin Williams, Billy Crystal, and several other entertainers who make it okay to visualize a chicken heart eating Chicago, or a kid named Fat Albert flattening a whole Buck Buck team, or a Valley Girl, or a silly old man on a park bench.

Audiences love to use their imaginations in settings where it is permissible. It becomes the job of the therapeutic facilitator to convince clients that it is also okay to have an image of a very wise old physician who lives inside them—a physician who can become present in any form they may choose. This Inner Physician may show itself as a dove, a lump of coal, an angel, or anything else. It is also possible that the Inner Physician may not present itself visually at all. It may present as a voice, a smell, or a feeling. However a client's Inner Physician chooses to present itself, the person must be helped to understand that this wise being can provide good advice; it knows and understands the problems; and it can be of inestimable help in finding solutions.

Clients must also be brought to understand that, if done carefully and politely, a dialogue can be established between their Inner Physician, their conscious awareness, and the therapeutic facilitator. Once the facilitator speaks directly to a person's Inner Physician, the option is available to keep the conversation confidential and not immediately available to the client's conscious awareness. I do this only at the request of the Inner Physician, however, or if it occurs spontaneously.

Amazingly, a symptom such as a back pain may be asked to present itself. Upon my request, my own chronic back pain presented itself as a boomerang. It spoke with me and told me about itself and its purpose. It told me that it only hurt me when it was inflated, and what inflated it was anger. It led me to understand that anger will always come back at me like a boomerang and give me back pain. I understood. Now when I have that back pain, I search inside to see what I'm angry about. When I find it and discharge it, the pain leaves. It is amazing how often we humans are subliminally angry. I thank my boomerang for letting me know.

This productive use of imagination, creativity, imagery, and internal dialogue flies in the face of what so many of us have been taught and conditioned to believe. We are conditioned to "get real" and "stay real." As a result, the most difficult part of therapeutic imagery and dialogue may be initiating it and making it credible. The therapeutic facilitator has to be a good salesperson in this instance. To sell, you must believe in your product. If therapists prove during training to be embarrassed, inhibited or skeptical of the efficacy of therapeutic imagery and dialogue, it is necessary to have someone work with them until they are comfortable with its concepts and uses. They will often require constant and literal reassurance and support as to the significance and credibility of what they are doing. This reassurance can be through words, tone of voice, touch, and intention. These modes may be used concurrently, interchangeably and individually as they seem appropriate at any given moment in any given session.

What's Quantum Physics Got to Do With It?

Quantum physics is the outgrowth of the seed planted by Max Planck in about 1900. It was around this time that he proposed the quantum theory: the concept that there is no such thing as a pure continuum in the physical world. Energy, motion and mass all exist in tiny parcels or "quanta," which only give the appearance of continuity because they are so small. When viewed in minute detail, however, all things are made up of tiny pieces.

For example, an oscillator does not gain or lose energy along a continuum. It gains or loses its energy in discrete amounts. Each quantum has a specific amount of energy. In electromagnetic radiation, the quantum is the photon.

In 1905 Einstein used Planck's quantum theory to explain the photoelectric effect. In 1913 Niels Bohr used Planck's theory to explain the atomic spectra. In 1933 Erwin Schrödinger was awarded the Nobel Prize for the development of the wave equation, which gave birth to quantum mechanics as it is today. Quantum mechanics is the science that describes electron and small particle behavior. Quantum electrodynamics is a further extension that deals with the behavior of charged particles in a quantized field. It is used to explain interactions between electrons, positrons and radiation. As far as I know, all of the quantum sciences are the progeny of Max Planck's insight that led him to the formulation of the quantum theory. What's quantum theory and quantum physics got to do with imagery and dialogue? We'll see.

From 1960 through 1964 I had the distinct privilege of working as a teaching and research fellow for a very brilliant man named Stacy F. Howell. He was a biochemist, and I was his first and only fellow. He was near retirement, so he used me as a sounding board for many thoughts and ideas he had developed during his lifetime. Dr. Howell had a huge stack of handwritten notes on the subject of size. He proposed as food for thought that a molecule may be a mini model of a galaxy, and an atomic nucleus might be a mini model of a sun with the electrons analogous to the planets circling that sun. He further proposed that these analogous relationships existed between all things; the only variable was size. He proposed that each particle was a hologram of the whole of which that particle was a fragment. He lectured to me and at me for hours on this subject. The cell was a mini human being and the electron was a mini earth circling its nucleus as earth circles the sun.

Letting our imaginations stretch a little, we can consider electrons and their possible analogous relationships to people, minds, imaginations, and images. When electrons are shot from electron guns, as in your television set, they seem able to behave as either particles or waves. For example, when we fire electrons through a slit into a cloud chamber, they seem to behave as particles. That is, they travel through the mist inside the chamber and leave a trail visible to the human observer. On the other hand, if we shoot electrons through the same slit at a photographic film, the results suggest that waves are striking the film. Thus begins the debate whether electrons are particles or waves.

This apparent discrepancy regarding the nature of the electron raises the question in the minds of some theoretical physicists as to whether the electron might be both a particle and a wave, depending on how we choose to observe it. The next question is whether the electron would behave as a particle or a wave, or neither of the two, if there were no observer. Perhaps the electron has a consciousness that understands our puzzlement and our need to understand. The electron may wish to accommodate us. Thus, if we decide to look for a particle, the electron acts like a particle. Or, if we are looking for a wave, it gives us a wave.

Sometimes electrons may be in a playful or contrary mood and behave in an opposite way from what we expect. It seems to happen fairly often that one experiment's results are opposite from another's. Are electrons mini people? Some show you what you want to see and others, being contrary, show you just the opposite of what you expect. If electrons are performing for the experimenter in the way the experimenter expects them to perform, what are the electrons doing when no experiment is in progress? Is there an electron behavioral phenomenon when no one is watching? Or does our watching trigger the behavior?

When we perceive something with our hands, is it still there even when our hands aren't there to perceive it? I have had many therapist/facilitators tell me about new rhythms they perceive and new vectors they see. It is both astonishing and sobering. Would these rhythms and vectors be there without the therapeutic facilitator? This sounds like imagination. It also sounds like I am making a case against the credibility of what hands-on therapists perceive. Not so. The amazing thing is that these imagined rhythms and vectors are often used successfully to obtain a positive therapeutic effect.

As I discussed these questions during a class in the spring of 1989, one of the participants described her experience. She had encountered some difficulty in using and seeing the vector/axis system as I had presented it. Being an impulsive, uninhibited, creative type, she invented her own vectors and axes. She invented a vector to serve whatever purpose she felt she needed. Lo and behold her imagined/invented/improvised vectors worked for her and her client. A positive therapeutic result was obtained. She stated that she had repeated this process many times with a very high percentage of success. I believed her.

When I and other therapeutic facilitators work with patients, we may get what we expect or we may get just the opposite. Just as there may be contrary electrons, there may be contrary people who give contrary responses. If we expect to feel the craniosacral system, we'll feel it. If we expect the manipulation of this craniosacral system to yield a positive therapeutic effect, it will—except in the case of a contrary response.

If we can get an image with the patient of what we truly and mutually want, we can have our wish. Perhaps reality occurs—with electrons and with people—when we perceive it. If this is true, when we image something, we make it happen. Used correctly, therapeutic imaging with dialogue is an extremely effective therapeutic modality.

That's what quantum physics has to do with it.

The Therapeutic Image

The therapeutic image may present itself either spontaneously (if there is such a thing) or upon the therapist's request. In either case, when a significant image presents itself to the client, the significance detector—the sudden stoppage of the craniosacral rhythm—will indicate that it has done so.

When a therapist is just working—there is no conversation or following of body position going on—and the craniosacral rhythm suddenly stops, this is the significance detector. It could stop during any phase of the pulse. It will often stop when there is an extreme degree of tension held in the system. This is in contrast to the relaxed state of the craniosacral system when a still point occurs.

The Unsolicited Image

When this sudden stop occurs, it means that something good is happening inside, and whatever it is has either arrived in the patient's conscious awareness or is just outside the boundary and is about to enter. The instant I feel the "stop," I might ask the patient, "What is in your mind right now?" I tell the individual not to worry about how silly it may seem and to just tell me what was there at the instant I asked the question. The patient usually has some difficulty answering. It may be like a dream, gone from awareness in a fraction of a second. It is a little like playing musical chairs. The music stops and you awkwardly scramble for a chair. With practice, however, you get better. Soon, when the music stops, you know precisely where you are in relation to each chair. The same is true with clients and the significance detector. Initially they may not be able to say what is going on at the precise instant they are asked, but with practice they will improve. It is very important for the therapist to be kind and let the client know that it is common for the instantaneous content to escape.

I often explain the significance detector to patients at this point. I tell them that the nonconscious may be bringing into awareness something that could be helpful; that I am able to pick this up as a signal from their bodies; and that I will repeat the question when I pick up the signal again. Now the nonconscious mind of the patient has heard my comments. It also has tentatively offered the tip of the iceberg. I am telling the nonconscious that I am ready to receive its message and would it please try to communicate with me. I suspect that these verbally unsolicited messages begin to come through because the non-

> ### Significance Detector
> The significance detector is the spontaneous cessation of the craniosacral rhythm. It is used to tell the SER practitioner whether or not a word, thought, or body position is significant. It is the same phenomenon as still point, except it occurs spontaneously during SER rather than through induction by the practitioner.

conscious part of the patient senses my touch and the open, helping, sincere attitude it conveys. The nonconscious part tentatively projects toward me with the hope that I am as sympathetic as my touch seems to be and that the healing process may develop.

After a few times of not being able to say what is in their minds at the specific instant when the question is asked, most people will begin to come up with something. This may not be a visual image. It may be a voice, a feeling, or a sense that "something" is there. I have had several cases where the initial unsolicited image was the smell of ether. Most patients have to be encouraged to speak about this sensation because they think it is silly and not what I am looking for. But if I follow this olfactory perception, it will usually lead into the reprocessing of a previous surgical experience.

The olfactory image of ether has very often come up with adults over fifty years old who are going back to reprocess a tonsillectomy. They often have to deal with issues of desertion by parents, impending death by breathing ether through a mask, assault by a doctor, or being lied to about the pain and therefore feeling betrayed. Each case is very individual, but many people initially seem to enter the process by smelling ether. It is not rare for the therapeutic facilitator to smell ether right along with the client as the experience and its attendant feelings unfold.

When this initial, unsolicited image presents itself, and the client is able to hold onto some part of it, the therapist must do everything in his or her power to help maintain contact with the part of the nonconscious that is presenting this image.

I softly and gently try to get the patient to provide more details about the image. With each detail the communication line is opened further. The rapport is strengthened between me, the patient's conscious awareness, and the nonconscious part that has made the initial communication gesture. I ask about size, shape, color, odor, sound, texture—anything I can think to ask will strengthen the rapport between conscious and nonconscious. I ask the patient how he or she feels in the presence of this image. I encourage the process with soft, simple urgings such as "go on" and "tell me more." One of my favorites is, "I'm not sure I understand. Can you help me to understand better what it is that you mean?" This lets patients know that I am really trying; it helps to dispel the usually troublesome therapist-patient hierarchy; and it really makes them part of the process, i.e., it suggests that they know something you don't.

Above all I try to be there with patients as they further describe their imaging experience. I blend and meld with them through my hands. I image to myself what they describe. The more I can see what they see, smell what they smell, hear what they hear, feel what they feel, and sense what they sense in every way possible, the more effectively the therapeutic process will progress.

Soliciting an Image

There are many ways to solicit an image. The client or the therapeutic facilitator can ask that an Inner Physician, an inner advisor, an inner wisdom, a higher self, a pain, a disease, a tumor, or anything else please come into conscious awareness and communicate. I like for the patient to use the plural pronoun "us" right from the start because it opens the door for the therapeutic facilitator to be included in the process from the beginning. Later, then, when I may wish to dialogue directly with the image, I am already at least partially accepted.

When I ask an image to present itself, my patient must be clear that it may assume a totally unexpected form. It is best to have no expectation. The patient must be continually reassured that any and every image is important; none is silly. The patient must be encouraged to describe whatever occurs. As the facilitator, I have the significance detector working for me. When "we" make a request for an image to communicate or come forward, I simply wait quietly until the cranio-sacral rhythm abruptly stops. When it does, I ask the individual what is there and what is sensed. (You know something is there, you just have to get the patient to tell you about it.)

If the patient begins to describe an image and the craniosacral rhythm has not stopped, I recognize that this is probably not a significant image. But I DO NOT, I repeat, DO NOT say that to the patient. I encourage him or her to work with this image for awhile. When I encounter this kind of resistance, I go with it. I don't set up an adversarial situation. I repeat my request or take a little rest. I might begin again with a new and different request.

After a few non-significant trials, an image that stops the craniosacral rhythm will usually occur. If not, it may be best to just do bodywork for the rest of that session and wait until the next visit to try imagery again. One has to be patient, working within the client's ground rules as much as possible. Above all, I don't impose my wishes and expectations on the patient.

Another possibility is that, as I pursue the non-significant image, the significance detector will suddenly tell me that something important has just come up and I need to follow it. This sometimes feels as though the patient's nonconscious is testing my sincerity.

Once I establish the image's presence, I begin the dialogue. At first I like to simply chat with the image, get friendly, and let the image get to know me. I want to help the image feel at ease. For example, I might say, "Hi, my name is John. I'm trying to help [the patient's name] get a handle on [the problem]. I would really like to talk with you. I have a feeling that you are really smart and could help us understand what is going on. I would like to be your friend, so perhaps you could tell me a name that you would prefer to be called." Image tells you its name. "That's a neat name. Have we met before?" I ask the image how long it has been aware of the problem, what it does, and so on. I really give the image a chance to express itself. I must be sincerely and genuinely interested. I try to find out what the image would like, what it might suggest, what it knows about the patient, and why the problem is there.

If I am talking with a symptom, I need to find out if it is happy doing what it is doing. The symptom is usually not happy, so I try to find out what would make it happy. Typically the symptom wants to be freed of the responsibility of being the symptom, but it feels an obligation to continue as an active symptom as long as the patient doesn't understand the problem or is unwilling to work toward its resolution.

Now I must get the patient to be aware of the purpose behind the symptom and demonstrate this awareness to the symptom. I must convince both patient and symptom that the patient will immediately begin working toward satisfactory resolution. Then I have to convince the symptom of the patient's sincerity and willingness to do this.

I may also have to educate the symptom. The symptom may not be aware that there is an alternative existence available for it. It thinks it has to make pain and is unable to do anything else. I let it know that if its purpose is accomplished and the patient changes, it can do something that is more fun, something that makes it happy. I might even present this happiness as a reward for good work. Symptoms may not have any idea what "happy" is, so I may have to help them understand.

Further, the symptom may not understand the impact that it is having on the patient's life. I may need to discuss whether the "punishment fits the crime." Frequently the symptom doesn't realize that the punishment is excessively severe. An example might be—and I have seen this quite often—severe pelvic pain in an adult woman that interferes with normal sexual activity. The pain (symptom) is punishment for fondling her genitalia as an infant or toddler. She may have been told repeatedly that good girls don't do such things. I only have to point out to the symptom that as a child the patient was only doing something that produced a pleasant sensation. She did not yet have a judgment and moral code about such things. Why, then, was the symptom still punishing her so severely thirty years later? I may have to reiterate this rationale a few times, but the symptom will usually agree at some point that the punishment has been excessively severe and is now inappropriate, or at least that the punishment has been sufficient and can stop now. At that juncture I can probably get the symptom to put its energy into a more constructive project of its own choosing—one that I, of course, will help it choose.

Tumors

Tumors present a special case for SomatoEmotional Release and Therapeutic Imagery and Dialogue because they can be deadly and frequently invoke great fear. I have had conversations with many tumors, although there were a few I just couldn't engage in a decent conversation. In general, the significant tumor will talk to you if you are gentle, respectful and persuasive. The insignificant tumor is often incommunicative and will not talk to you. The Inner Physician may let you know, however, that this tumor is not significant and therefore does not have much to say.

Significant tumors can be either malignant or benign. In either case they want to be heard, so I solicit their dialogue. Malignant tumors may be aware that they are deadly but see no way out. Or they may not be aware (or pretend they aren't aware) that continuation of their present activity may be deadly to the host. If the host dies, so does the tumor. I make this fact perfectly clear to the tumor. Sometimes the tumor thinks it will go on living even if the host dies. In many of these cases I have to introduce the tumor to the real world. I may be able to introduce alternatives to death, even if the tumor feels all is hopeless.

I worked with a tumor a few years ago that had to be convinced it would die when the host died. The tumor, which was a breast cancer, was convinced it had tried to get the patient to change her lifestyle but had failed in this task; therefore, the tumor reasoned, the woman would be better off dead than alive. The tumor informed me that when its host died it would just move on to someone else who needed "guidance." I had to convince the tumor it would cease to exist if the patient died. It would not just go into someone else's body to repeat its cycle.

I also had to convince the tumor that the host did not know what it was trying to tell her. She did not know she was supposed to change her lifestyle, nor did she know in what way her lifestyle should be changed. The "crime" was a rejection of femininity. I took the stance that death was a severe punishment for such a crime. I had to explain fun and happiness to this tumor and convince it that, if it would lighten up and allow the patient some time to change, it could perhaps find a happier existence.

I asked the tumor to regress immediately because of the threat to life it posed. The tumor agreed to regress (shrink, involute) while it watched to see if the host would really change lifestyles. The host did, and the tumor became no longer diagnosable by traditional medical methods. When I dialogued afterward with the tumor, it said it was still there as a seed and could recur any time this patient deviated from the new and acceptable lifestyle. Now the patient and her tumor dialogue every morning, so if deviations from what the tumor considers "acceptable" happen, I'm sure there will be negotiation between the tumor and host before dangerous regrowth occurs.

This same patient has cystic mastitis of both breasts. Her Inner Physician says these multiple benign tumor growths are not of any real significance. She can image them away if she wants to. It makes no difference to her Inner Physician. She is working on the normalization of her cystic fibrotic breast tissue for her comfort and self-esteem, not because this tissue has any deep meaning in her life.

Another example of insignificant tumors occurred in a sixty-seven-year-old man who had been doing some very successful therapeutic imagery with his heart. During a routine physical exam he was found to have multiple colon polyps, and surgery was scheduled. During one of his visits with me he asked if we could do anything about the polyps. I suggested we could always explore the possibilities.

We connected with his Inner Physician who told us that the polyps lacked any particular purpose. They just happened because he repeatedly ate and drank substances in the past that irritated his bowel. He did not do these things anymore, but the lining of his bowel had become chronically irritated over the years. Mucus production had inordinately increased, and the bowel lining had separated from the underlying muscular wall in several places. Polyps formed at these sites of separation. I asked if we could do anything to avoid the necessity for surgical removal and if this would be acceptable. The Inner Physician said for us to go ahead and heal the polyps by focusing a healing light and energy in the bowel.

I placed my hands in front and back of the supine patient's body with the sigmoid colon between them. We mutually conjured up a generic healing-light energy. The energy accumulated and enlarged in magnitude. The light kept changing color. We both saw this simultaneously. Then the energy dissipated suddenly and the light softened. We knew the work was accomplished.

The patient went for surgery about three weeks later. The surgeon put in the sigmoidoscope and, to his bewilderment, there were no colon polyps to be found. This case is an example of benign tumors with no particular significance in the patient's present life. They were simply remnants of his previous lifestyle. I would not attempt this process without permission from the patient's Inner Physician!

Emotions

SomatoEmotional Release is part of the bigger picture of the role of emotions in health and life in general. Conversely, an understanding of the role of emotion is necessary to understand SER. The therapeutic images that appear in dialogue with the Inner Physician often show the patient as being stuck in a particular emotional posture.

It has been fairly common in my experience to find a patient literally full to the brim with potentially destructive emotions such as anger, hate, guilt, fear, resentment, jealousy, or any combination thereof. I can usually feel these emotions as soon as I touch a patient. Sometimes I am hit in the face with them when I enter the treatment room, sometimes even before I enter the room.

I used to think that it was best to discharge destructive emotions immediately and then look for causes. The next phase would be to focus on turning off their production by resolving the problem. More recently, it dawned on me that the energy which comprises these destructive emotions is the same energy that makes up such constructive emotions as love, joy and hope. It therefore seems logical that, in order to conserve a patient's energy and enhance his or her self-esteem, it is preferable to convert destructive emotion into constructive emotion.

Now I usually ask the patient's Inner Physician whether it would be possible and preferable to perform the conversion. When the answer is yes—as seems to be the case about fifty or sixty percent of the time—I proceed along this line, getting as much advice and direction as I can from the Inner Physician. When the answer is, "No, let's just get it out of here," or words to that effect, I most often use my hands to help in the release or extraction process.

Usually I have the patient localize the destructive emotion under my hands. Together we imagine that my hands are magnets that can draw the destructive emotion out of the person's body. I used to have patients push hard from the inside, but I have come to realize that less physical effort on their part often facilitates the therapeutic process. Now I try to establish a "let it go" rather than a "push it out" attitude.

Before I describe the actual release and extraction process, there are two further issues I want to clarify. Number one, I like to explain to patients that as soon as the destructive emotion passes out of their bodies, we will neutralize it and have it converted to generic energy that can be used for constructive purposes by whomever might need it. This precautionary step serves to allay any concerns they may have about polluting the atmosphere if destructive energy is let out of their bodies. I have found that many people fall back on martyrdom and convince themselves that it is better to keep the bad stuff rather than release it into the world where it can damage other unsuspecting and innocent victims. You can defuse this line of defense by neutralizing the destructive energy as it leaves the body.

Number two, I like to explain to patients that they do not have to physically act upon the destructive energy as they feel it localize and release. For example, if we are discharging anger, I simply let these patients know that they will feel angry as the energy precipitates, localizes, and concentrates in the selected area of the body in preparation for release. I let them know that this anger can go directly out through their skin into the atmosphere. It does not have to be acted upon by kicking, screaming, beating on me, or trashing my treatment room. They can just let it go. As it releases, they will feel the emotion diminish and disappear.

At this point I probably should explain why I use the words "destructive" and "constructive" to describe the various emotions we all feel. I used to describe emotions as "negative" and "positive." Anger, hatred, jealousy, fear, and resentment were negative. Joy, love, hope, serenity, and the like, were positive. I have encountered some confusion using "negative" and "positive." The negatives were undesirable and the positives were desirable emotions in my view. However, we might also discuss a negatively charged electrical atmosphere that is desirable for good health and function, or an accumulation of positive ions in an airplane cabin, which is detrimental. So to avoid confusion, I am using "destructive" and "constructive."

Facilitators-in-training frequently baulk at this point, saying, "Wait a minute, anger isn't necessarily destructive. It may save your life in an emergency or help you survive later when you need energy to keep going." This is true. Anger might give you the superhuman strength to cripple Hulk Hogan were he to attack you. But when this anger continues, it becomes destructive. Anger is a spender. It demands of your heart, your lungs, your liver, your stomach, your colon, your entire physiology. It allows no quarter for the replacement of what it takes from you. It works just like the sympathetic nervous system. It will save your life in an emergency and keep you going under stress, but it will also hasten your demise. It is destructive when the emergency is over and your life has been spared. Hate, anger, jealousy, fear, and guilt will consume and destroy their owner if they maintain an ongoing residence.

I have also heard the argument that guilt and fear contribute to the formation of conscience and are therefore "good emotions." True, guilt and fear (of punishment) may prevent you from robbing a bank, stealing a car, embezzling from your boss, or killing your spouse's lover. Still, it is much healthier—both physically and emotionally—if you do not commit wrongful acts because you love and respect humanity, because you are understanding rather than vengeful, and because you can tolerate a reasonable amount of unpleasantness at the hands of others. None of us is perfect. We all need to understand this as we strive to improve.

Please tolerate my tendency to sermonize. It just seems more appropriate at this time to describe emotions as destructive and constructive rather than negative or positive. I doubt that I have to justify to you readers the idea that happiness, joy, hope, serenity, and the like, are constructive to the whole being.

While on the subject of destructive emotion, I would like to share two experiences and how they contributed to my evolving concept of fear and its relation to anger and guilt.

I was on the massage table going through a SomatoEmotional Release. The process was part of an ongoing saga that had begun several years earlier. I had already established that, shortly after my birth, my mother would often go into a rage at my presence. At the time I believed I was an unwanted nuisance. Yet it wasn't until this SER experience that I understood the error of this assumption.

The abusive treatment began when I was three days old. I learned quickly that to cry or make noise invited even more pain. If I attracted attention when my diapers were dirty, for instance, I might end up suspended by my ankles while my skin was scrubbed hard. I even remember developing pneumonia at three months old. I could actually visualize it in my right lung. But if I coughed and made noise, I'd get hurt by my mother; so I learned how "to breathe around" the infected area. I was becoming a master at rejecting the fear response, maintaining control, becoming invisible. All I needed to survive was a keen awareness.

I know this all sounds brutal, but during my SER session I came to know that my mother, my sister, my maternal grandfather, and I were "of the same spirit." We were sent down by a soul to teach each other the lessons for which we were earthbound. My grandfather taught me about street wisdom. My sister, who has always been there for me, taught me about love. And my mother? She taught me to be wary of danger without being afraid. Since then I've encountered many potentially intimidating situations traveling the path laid out for me. For me to do what I've had to do in this lifetime, I could not have been controlled by fear. Fortunately, I was a quick learner. By the time I was four years old, the rages and abuse stopped.

Perhaps you can understand why I've never been angry with my mother. Instead I feel compassion. I recognize that she must have been mentally off-balance during the first years of my life. Without reservation, I accept that she was teaching me not to be victimized by fear.

I recall being seriously afraid only twice later in my life: once as a child faced with a bully toting a BB gun, and later as a young adult, when I was the only medical personnel onboard a Coast Guard cutter rescuing eleven men whose tugboat had sunk two hundred miles out in the Gulf of Mexico. Those occasions only reinforced my lessons. I have never again allowed fear to paralyze my brain.

Several weeks after that SER, with all my realizations still fresh, I was working with a Vietnam veteran during a ten-day intensive treatment program for post-traumatic stress disorder (PTSD). This particular vet was an ex-marine who lied about his age and was sent at age sixteen to Vietnam, where he became a brainwashed, highly trained killer. He carried a machine gun with instructions to shoot anything that moved. He said he killed several people nearly every day for a year.

During our sessions he began to see the faces of people he shot. Suddenly he realized that many had been civilians, even women and children. That's when he began confronting the conflict between his survival skills and his conscience, between his orders and his guilt at having followed them.

His body shook as he vacillated between rage and remorse. As I blended with him, it became clear that his fear had motivated his violent activities. In order to create a killer, his military trainers had implanted a deep fear in him for his own life. Yet I also sensed a natural compassion that had been held at bay by fear and was now fueling his inner war. To end that war, we would need to either neutralize or discharge the fear.

Let me tell you a little more about how fear affected this man. Prior to our program, he called to tell us not to pick him up at the airport as arranged. He wouldn't be on the flight because he couldn't control his fear of flying. He would come by train instead, even though it was a fifteen-hour ride. The person who finally showed up put on a tough, skeptical image. He had a short, G.I. haircut plus a mustache and goatee. His eyes shifted from flat and emotionless to piercing and threatening in seconds. He let us know he was a loner. Never married. Trusted only one or two people in the world. Yet his lean body responded well to our first days of compassionate CranioSacral Therapy and touch.

Then we came to the seventh day of our program. The part of his nervous system that responded to danger—the reticular alarm system (RAS)—was set on ready alert. He was literally poised for combat at the sound of a pin dropping or the sensation of anything threatening or unfamiliar. Put simply, it was the sort of stress that triggered his trained behavior. We could see he had to work hard to control his "killer" reflexes.

Sensing his inner wisdom, I explained that his RAS was still hyperactive from his experiences in Vietnam. I also explained that this was at least partially responsible for his post-traumatic stress disorder and its disabling effects—that is, his inability to live comfortably in the social structure surrounding him. All this was done, of course, while numerous therapeutic facilitators assisted him.

I then asked permission to dialogue directly with whatever body parts might help us to better understand the problems he was suffering. He agreed, so I asked the RAS to speak with me through the vet. RAS told me it was too busy focusing on its job. I asked how long it had been since it had been relaxed. RAS said it didn't know—it may never have been relaxed. So I asked the amygdalae (the parts of the brain in command of emotional responses) if they were in charge of RAS's activity. They said RAS was out of their control and had been for a long time.

I asked our vet to visualize a gauge from 0 to 100 that represented his RAS activity level. He cooperated, visualizing the kind of gauge that is common on oxygen tanks. His RAS was running at 80. I again explained how this level probably helped save his life in Vietnam but could be harmful now. I asked if he would be willing to lower the reading to 50, which he did. As he reported his progress, we felt his tissues relax. We soon sensed his fluid and energy flow improve, as well.

Then I asked him to try for 25. He got the gauge down to 20 but began to experience severe back and chest pain. The gauge spontaneously returned to 50 and the pain left. When he forced the gauge below 50 again the pain returned.

This pattern repeated several times until it became clear that the pain was the voice of something inside him that didn't want the RAS activity to go down. So I asked "Pain" about the situation. It said it was dangerous for the vet to relax his guard; he could be killed.

After some conversation we realized that fear controlled the RAS activity level. It was responsible for our veteran's inability to embark on a post-war healing process. The fear felt justified in its actions, however, since it was responsible for the vet's survival in Vietnam. The problem was, it didn't realize the war was over.

Suddenly I saw how my own experiences with my mother could

help me here. I learned that you can be alert to danger without using fear as the stimulating mechanism. Fear actually reduces the effectiveness with which we respond to danger.

I shared this with our veteran. He understood. His RAS liked the idea of not being driven by fear. His amygdalae were overjoyed. Yet "Fear" was totally unreasonable, so it had to be forcibly removed. That involved a lot of strong therapist "intention" along with a few therapeutic surprises. In any case, the fear suddenly discharged, the pain left, and the RAS gauge dropped to 20, where I'm pleased to say it remained.

This story has a happy ending. Our veteran, at his own suggestion, flew home. He called us after his safe return to proudly tell us his flight was uneventful. He experienced no fear.

Acupuncture and the Emotions

Clinical observation and experience has demonstrated to my satisfaction that specific emotions accumulate in specific body organs. Specific organ-emotion associations agree in large part with concepts put forth in traditional Chinese literature and acupuncture. My first exposure to the idea that specific organs collect and store excesses of specific emotions came in 1968 when I began studying acupuncture literature. I was very skeptical, but somehow my mind remained open to the possibility. (I can't take credit for this openness on a conscious level, but somehow it was there.) Over the years I have come to trust the acupuncture system of diagnosis and treatment. Later in this book I will share the experience that led me to this confidence.

In traditional Chinese medicine, specific body organs are associated with specific emotions. As I have suggested, organs in acupuncture are not exactly the same as they are in our Western physiology. The organs include not only the physical heart, lungs, kidneys, and so forth, but the type of chi energy associated with them and the "meridians" or "channels" along which that energy flows. Chi flows from the organ through the body to the surface, where the meridian terminates at the ends of the fingers or toes, or from the terminating points towards the organ. The chi of the organs can be accessed through specific points along the meridians by the insertion of needles (acupuncture) or other means, such as the application of manual pressure (acupressure) or the burning of special substances over the points (moxibustion).

The organs and their meridians are characterized as yin or yang, and the chi in the body is also yin and yang. Health in general is identified as having a proper yin/yang balance, and diagnosis and treatment efforts attempt to restore yin/yang imbalances.

The meridians are named according to the organ systems with which they are associated. The points along the meridians are numbered in sequence according to the direction the chi energy is said to flow. Thus, "Liver 3" is the third point along the liver meridian. The condition of a given organ system can be felt by palpating the pulses along the meridians.

Since traditional Chinese medicine associates the organs with specific emotional qualities, any deficiencies or excesses in the energy of a given organ may express themselves as imbalances in the emotional life of the client. In this way treatment by acupuncture integrates physical symptoms with emotional qualities. The process of SomatoEmotional Release is often enhanced by working with the acupuncture meridians that correspond to the emotions that are crying out to be released.

I have found the following partial table of what we might call "visceroemotional" correspondences to be reliable. They keep showing up in patient after patient.

> Liver: anger and depression
>
> Heart: love and fear of being hurt emotionally
>
> Pericardium: protector of the heart
>
> Lungs: grief
>
> Kidneys: fear of death
>
> Spleen: disappointment

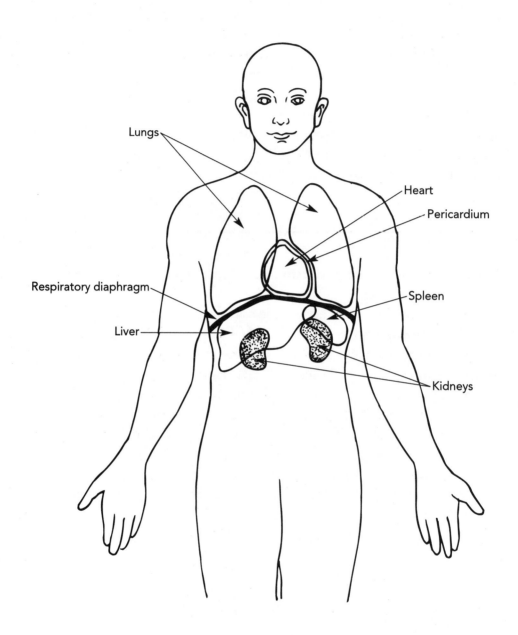

Illustration 4-1.

The Liver

The liver collects, stores, and is the seat of anger and depression. The first time I really became convinced of this relationship was when I treated a patient in a psychiatric ward. She had made three apparently valid but unsuccessful attempts at suicide. She was in depression so deep that speaking was an effort, moving was seldom voluntary, and, to be honest, I could hardly see her breathe. Her skin color was yellowish-white and transparent. I could feel the hopelessness of this poor woman as soon as she entered my space. She was about sixty years old and had been divorced for twenty years when I met her. She had fallen into this depression about ten years before when an air crash killed her son. She came to see me with her sister, who had obtained permission from the psychiatrist for a day pass.

Her liver felt like a bowling ball in both size and consistency. It felt like it weighed about twenty pounds. I put my hands on the front and back of her body so that the liver was between them. She was supine on the treatment table. Attempting to release her liver in this way was like trying to dissolve a bowling ball with my hands.

I decided to use acupuncture for her depression in accordance with Felix Mann's recipe from his book *Acupuncture: Treatment of Many Diseases*. I put needles in acupuncture points along her liver meridian on both sides of her body. I went back to her liver with my hands and could feel it begin to soften and respond much more readily to my passage of energy through it.

As the liver softened and released, I felt energy forces come from her skin in the front, back and right side where the skin overlays the liver. Her breathing deepened visibly; her color changed from yellowish-white to pinkish-white; she began to move voluntarily a little; and her face began to show traces of transient expressions. In short, she started looking less like a jaundiced zombie and more like an uncomfortable human who still had some fight left in her. I stayed with the liver until its release seemed complete. I did not dialogue with her, but I kept up a constant patter of encouragement in my mind. I was silently urging her to let it go.

After her liver had softened and released the heavy, heavy energy that I assume was her depression, she got a little feisty. She complained about the needles and how long everything was taking. I then went to her craniosacral system and released the compression that was present above her sacrum, at the base of her skull, and elsewhere. When she left, you could hardly tell she was depressed. Mostly she was angry and complaining about everything.

I saw this woman on two more occasions at weekly intervals. I did additional manual release of the energy of anger from her liver. No further acupuncture was used. I treated the craniosacral system. She was discharged from the hospital after her second visit with me because she had a "spontaneous remission" of her depression. (Her sister did not tell the psychiatrist that I was treating her when she took her out on the day passes.) By the third visit she had stopped taking all her medications. She remained fine for six months after our final session, and I have not heard from her or her sister since.

This experience made me consider that perhaps the major depressive shock of the sudden and surprising loss of this woman's son had been absorbed into her liver. Her liver was overwhelmed by the size of the shock. It became a seat of anger at the fates for taking her son from her. It also became a seat of despondency because there was nothing she could do about the death. Since the liver could not handle it all, it then became the ongoing source of the continuing depressive energy and underlying anger that contaminated her whole emotional being. I liken the liver to the oil filter in a car. This filter acts as an oil cleanser until the filter cartridge is full, then it becomes a source of dirt in the oil of your car's engine. If you drain the dirty oil and put in clean oil but do not install a new oil filter, the dirty filter cartridge soon contaminates your new, fresh, clean oil. Perhaps this is what psychotherapy does for depression: It puts in clean energy, but if the liver filter isn't cleansed or released, it constantly recontaminates the emotional being with depressive and angry energy.

The Heart

The heart is the filter, seat and storage bin of the fear of being hurt by loving someone who may not return your love or may desert you. An injured heart that is protecting itself against such an experience will not allow its owner to give unconditional love. The owner of this protecting heart fears entering a true, loving relationship and is afraid of getting hurt again. Some of this fear may be valid, but life without a true love relationship is an empty life indeed. It seems that to really love we have to trust the person we love. This represents a risk that some people are not willing or able to take. These people may rationally want to love but are emotionally unable to do so.

The offer of conditional love—"I'll love you if you'll love me back"— is a sign that the fear in the heart needs to be released if the person wants to enter a full and satisfying love relationship. An interesting sign of this fear is the prenuptial agreement. It seems to say, "I love you, but I'm not sure, so just in case ..." When fear is released in such a person's heart, he or she may burn the prenuptial agreement.

We must also be aware that an unconditional love relationship does not necessarily have to be with a mate or of a sexual nature. It may be with a sibling, a parent, a friend, or anyone else. Unconditional love leads to accepting other people's imperfections as well as our own. Once we accept the imperfect state of humanity and have released the fear in our hearts, unconditional love for everyone can follow.

I worked as a therapeutic facilitator for about three years with a certain female politician. (I am taking liberties in describing her case in order to protect her identity.) She originally began to see me in order to discover why she was fifty pounds overweight and could not lose the weight. The more successful she became, the more weight she gained and the less successful she was at dieting.

A lot of deep work showed several contributing factors to the weight problem. Among them were remembrances as a tiny child of her grandmother who, as a successful national politician, frequently talked in the patient's presence about "throwing your weight around" in order to be a success in politics. She also used to say that one "had to be big enough to cast a shadow that could not be ignored." We also got into the idea that as an adolescent she had decided that being overweight was the only way to develop an ample bosom which would attract male admiration. When she went on a diet she lost breast tissue, which she felt deep in her heart was necessary in order to be an attractive female. The patient was in her forties when I worked with her. She had borne three children with an alcoholic husband. She had divorced him several years before deciding to become a professional politician.

All of these insights helped to rectify the weight problem to some extent. She was able to lose and keep off about twenty-five of the fifty unwanted pounds. Then a romantic episode came into her life. It was with the same man for whom she had wanted an ample bosom when she was about fourteen years of age and he was about twenty-four. She had thought at the time she needed breasts to get his attention. She was now deeply in love with him and he had proposed marriage. She discovered, however, that she was very afraid to answer yes. She created a multitude of logical reasons to be afraid, but she really wanted to love him and to be with him. Among her reasons to decline his proposal: He wanted to semi-retire and sail the Caribbean on his yacht. She wanted to keep moving upward with her political aspirations. What if he cheated on her? What if he fell out of love after awhile? What if, what if, what if?

Her heart felt like it was being squeezed—and it quite possibly was. The pericardium, which surrounds the heart, is the heart protector. It will frequently almost strangle the heart in an attempt to protect it from further injury. I knew that her heart was very fearful of becoming involved in unconditional love, and the pericardium was certainly doing a great job of insulating this fearful heart.

As we worked with imagery and dialogue toward release of the heart's fear, we came to a vivid memory from about the first three days of her postpartum life. Acting as a third-party observer, the patient described what happened. After she was cleaned following birth and her mother was recovered from the anesthesia, the new-born was brought in to be with her mother. She was put on her mother's breast, but nothing came as she suckled. This event recurred several times during the first few days after delivery. Her mother finally became exasperated and angry with herself. In her anger, her mother then rejected breastfeeding as a viable method of nurturing her child. The patient took the end of breastfeeding attempts as a per-sonal rejection. She accepted her mother's anger as being a result of something she had done.

During the first three days of her life, the patient's pattern was set. She was afraid to love unconditionally because she would be rejected again. After all, she had loved her mother. Her mother got mad at her and wouldn't give her mother's milk. The logic she developed went something like this: If you love, people see your faults; then they can leave you or reject you. A solid basis for fear of loving had been put into place during the first week of her life.

In addition—and I'm sure you can see it coming—the mother's feelings of breast inadequacy were broadcast to the infant. As our infant grew to adolescence, she was determined not to have the same inadequacies as her mother; therefore, if she had to get fat to get ade-quate breasts, that is exactly what she would do—and continue to do throughout her life.

Release of the pericardial shielding device and the grip of fear from this lady's heart impacted her life significantly. She dropped her "what ifs" and married the man she loved, with only minor trepida-tion. Since then she has done some cruising with him on his yacht and likes it better than she thought she might. She got out of politics after a few face-saving maneuvers. She seems happy, content, and deeply in love for the first time in her life. And she really trusts her husband. She is now vulnerable, but it seems that deep and magnif-icent rewards require risk. On the other hand, if you believe and trust, there is no risk because you know that all will be taken care of and work out for the best.

The Pericardium

The pericardium is the protector of the heart. When the heart has been hurt, the pericardium springs into action and shields it from further injury, as we have just seen. This is a wonderful defense mechanism, but it seems that the pericardium has a very powerful tendency to be overly protective once it is called into action. As a therapist, I cannot release the fear in the heart unless I release the pericardium, either at the same time or beforehand. The example just given clearly illustrates how well the heart and pericardium work in conjunction with each other. I have had hundreds of patients who demonstrated that there cannot be real unconditional love if the pericardium is busy protecting the heart.

I frequently use the pericardial meridian as a release valve in these cases. I most often connect with this meridian at the front surface of the wrist, where the meridian crosses the wrist's creases. I use this as a "sink" or drain for energy in the pericardium. I place one hand over the pericardium on the left side of the front of the chest. With the other hand, I place two or three fingers along the meridian at the wrist between the points designated P6 and P7 on Illustration 4-2. Then I imagine energy flowing from the chest to the wrist. Sometimes I cycle it back from the patient's wrist, through my body to the patient's chest, thus completing the loop. I do so when it feels appropriate. If I encounter stiff resistance in the meridian, I send the energy back and forth between my hands repeatedly, a few seconds in each direction. I keep doing this until the resistance wears down and the meridian feels open.

Once open, the pericardium can soften and relax. Sometimes I have to dialogue with the pericardium and try to convince it that the patient really wants it to relax so that he or she can experience the joy of unconditional love. I may have to discuss trust, risk, vulnerability, and so on. The patient may decide, along with the pericardium, not to take the risk. That is the individual's choice. The facilitator's

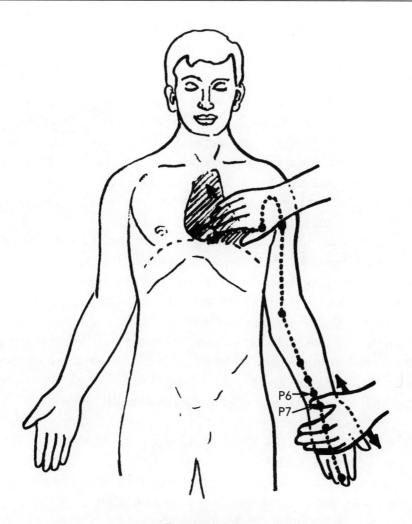

Illustration 4-2.
Shown is the pericardium (shaded), which protects the heart from further pain,
and the pericardial meridian through which pericardial restriction can be released.
See Text.

responsibility is to enlighten, not to force compliance with his or her views and opinions.

The Lungs

The lungs will serve as a filter, seat and storage organ for grief. It seems that the overloading of unresolved grief in the lungs is often an underlying cause for asthma, chronic bronchitis, respiratory allergies, shortness of breath for no apparent reason, and so on. Rib cages won't move right and diaphragms won't allow deep breathing. I also believe that some people use the narcotic effect of tobacco smoke to deaden the pain of grief in the lungs. (At some point in my career I would really like to test this hypothesis.)

There are numerous cases in our files that illustrate the release of grief from the lungs. This grief is identified as it passes through conscious awareness upon its release. An interesting patient I had the privilege of working with was a woman in her early thirties. She had developed asthma following the C-section delivery in her eighth month of a fetus who lived only a few hours. She kept a stiff upper lip because she did not want to emotionally injure her other children who were two and five years of age. She developed respiratory problems shortly after the delivery and was diagnosed as asthmatic.

Craniosacral evaluation with arcing gave the impression that, although the connective tissue in her upper body was not moving, no active lesion pathology was involved. The dural tube was also restricted through most of her body. When I placed my hands on her upper body, it felt like it was full of cement; it felt heavy like grief. Using SomatoEmotional Release and Therapeutic Imagery and Dialogue, we established the need to complete the delivery vaginally and to complete the grieving process—both in the lung tissues and emotionally. This was done and the asthma left as quickly as it came.

The Kidneys

The kidneys are often the filter, seat and storage organs for a very particular kind of fear, quite different from the heart's fear of being hurt. I call this fear the loss of immortality. By this I mean the fear that when you die, if you have no progeny, it's all over. One might the-orize that in order for the species to continue, each individual has an instinct to reproduce and thus achieve a sort of chromosomal immor-tality. Fear that you will not reproduce and thus continue your genetic lineage is filtered and stored in the kidneys.

This kind of problem is present in many men as they contemplate vasectomy and in women who are considering tubal ligation or hys-terectomy. It can be seen in parents awaiting grandparenthood if the process seems to be taking too long. It shows up in parents who endure the death of a child who has not yet reproduced. Women who have had miscarriages or abortions and have no living children will often demonstrate fear in the kidneys. These fears should be released from the kidneys. It will frequently require confrontation with the reality that there may be no progeny for any number of reasons.

Release of the fear usually is not too difficult, but the facilitator's skills may well be taxed as he or she tries to bring about acceptance of the situation as it is. The client's chromosomal future often has its end in sight, and this is not easily accepted. Recognition of the under-lying problem is mandatory. Acceptance and resolution are also nec-essary, or the kidneys will refill with fear. The fear-filled kidney shows itself as sexual dysfunction, recurrent bladder infections or inflam-mations, chronic anxiety, perfectionism, and high blood pressure.

A sixty-five-year-old man with whom I worked for several years suffered from chronic kidney dysfunction manifested by blood, albu-men, and uric acid crystals in the urine. He also suffered from severe heart disease and high blood pressure. He ultimately died of heart failure.

His course of declining health illustrates the role of fear in the kid-neys and the effect on total physiology. I was not able to get an accept-ance and resolution of the cause of the fear. His fear was well-founded. He was sixty-five and had never sired a child. As far as he was con-cerned, when he died his chromosomal or genetic lineage ended. He could not accept an eternal soul concept as a viable alternative. He really wanted his genes to be passed along.

The point of the case is that we were able periodically to empty the fear from his kidneys using SomatoEmotional Release and Therapeutic Imagery and Dialogue. He had weekly urine studies and daily blood pressure readings. He was well-monitored by internal medicine specialists in heart and kidney function. When his kidneys felt void of the cold, heavy energy, which I am calling fear, his urinalysis studies moved toward normal, his cardiac function improved, and his blood pressure normalized. These changes would last two or three weeks, then his test results and function would become abnormal again. We worked together over a period of five years and observed this roller-coaster effect probably ten times a year.

Each time we discharged the fear he rallied significantly, but we could never get past the idea that when he died his whole ancestral lineage went with him. He was an only child and felt the burden of responsibility to carry on his family name and the family genes. His parents had placed this burden on his shoulders very early in life, so death was not only scary, it was failure. The poor man died following a cardiac catheterization test that a new cardiologist convinced him he needed.

All cases are not so dreary, but one has to recognize that it often takes a powerful lot of talking and convincing to get barren patients past the fear that strikes when the end of their chromosomal lineage is in sight. If the outlook is not so bleak, it may be possible to help them see that all they need is a child or grandchild to keep their kidneys clear of the fear of loss of (genetic) immortality.

The Spleen

The spleen filters and stores disappointment of the type that results from observing "man's inhumanity to man." Probably the best example I can give of this type of splenic disappointment is my own rather dramatic experience. I was being treated by an Advanced CranioSacral Therapy class. In short order, attention was focused upon my spleen. I soon visualized a hollow bamboo tube coming straight up out of it, with a yellow liquid spilling from it onto the floor. As this occurred—and it seemed to last for an hour—I felt the sensation of my spleen deflating.

While this yellow liquid of disappointment was being forced from my spleen, I imaged a newsreel of the wars and atrocities that we humans do to one another: I saw Israelis and Arabs killing each other; I saw bombings and warlike activity in Northern Ireland; I saw the Falkland Islands war between Britain and Argentina; I saw us in Vietnam; and I saw the Crusaders killing people in the name of God.

Before this treatment, I could become livid with anger when I thought about our social injustices, unnecessary killing and massacres. I considered these things unforgivable and could almost give myself a stroke or heart attack just thinking about them. Since the release of the energy of disappointment from the spleen, I still feel badly about what we humans do to each other, but I am not so affected physiologically or emotionally by things I cannot immediately affect. I will still work against them, but the tremendous emotional upset does not accompany the knowledge. Now I simply accept that people have a lot more evolving to do before they will treat each other humanely. I now also know that people will never do what I want them to do, so I'm not so disappointed when they don't follow my rules.

Right Timing

In dialoguing with the Inner Physician, spokesperson or guide, I must always inquire as to how much I should tell the patient after he or she comes out of the deep relaxation state. I feel it is almost always necessary to bring the content of the session into the patient's conscious awareness. I will discuss this opinion with the nonconscious spokesperson or guide and try to point out the benefit. I like to make it a question of "when," not "if." Once this is accomplished, I gently try to bring the acceptable time of disclosure closer to the present. I try not to push too hard. I have had two lessons from patients that illustrate the importance of timing in revealing the content presented by the nonconscious.

Let's first consider the case of a twenty-four-year-old named Michael who came to my office in 1965 because he wanted to use hypnosis for weight reduction. He had seen me on a local broadcast of a medical panel discussion of various uses of hypnosis in anesthesia, as a behavior modifier, and as a means of accessing suppressed information, memories, feelings, and experiences. He was five feet, ten inches tall and weighed three hundred and twenty pounds. He stated that he had weighed over two hundred pounds in the eighth grade, and his eating and drinking of high-calorie sodas had been out of control for as long as he could remember. He had tried almost every diet he ever heard of and never lasted more than five to ten days on any of them. Appetite-suppressant pills made him so nervous that he could not use them. Michael was very ready to try hypnoregression to search for the psychoemotional reasons for his uncontrollable abuse of food and soft drinks. (He denied the use of alcohol.)

Michael was an excellent hypnotic subject and was induced into a deep trance during the first session. While he was in the trance, I had him discuss with me the reasons he wanted to lose weight. He told me he used his weight as a protection against being hurt. I asked him if he was willing to look for the reasons he needed the fat shield and if he would share those reasons with me. Michael's nonconscious agreed, and we began the regression.

I first asked Michael to go back to a happy time before he was fat. He went back to the fourth grade when he was on stage in a school spelling bee. He recalled the words and spelled them for me. He described the girl competing against him in the finals. Then he described her erroneous spelling of her word and how sorry he felt for her. But the sympathy was short-lived as he spelled the word correctly. He won! It felt wonderful!

Then it felt awful. The teacher in charge disqualified Michael, accusing him of cheating. After he had won the contest, he had taken a tiny piece of paper from his pocket that contained words used in the spelling bee. Michael denied looking at the paper while he spelled his words, explaining that the paper was how he studied. His appeals were to no avail, however, and he was disqualified.

He went to his grandmother's house after school because he was ashamed to face his mother. Grandma believed him. She fed him milk and cookies and cake and ice cream. She told him not to worry, she would protect him. Somehow he connected the food given him by Grandma with his protection against failure and the world's accusations. He began to eat for protection on that day and had been compulsively putting away excess calories ever since.

I brought Michael out of the trance slowly. As I did so, I instructed him that the next time we met he would go deeply into the special sleep where we could talk to his unconscious again. (I was saying "unconscious" in those days.) I also suggested that he would feel fine and rested when he awoke. I further let him know that he would remember only the details he could handle or deal with. Anything that was too much for him he could leave in his unconscious for the time being. Michael remembered nothing when he awoke. He felt fine. He asked a few innocuous questions and left the office.

He had three more weekly appointments, all of which were much the same as the first. We continued to identify the spelling bee episode as the initial cause for his need for protection, and his grandmother as the factor that started him using food as the preferred protection against the cruel world.

After each of the four weekly sessions, he had no recall of its content. He asked a few questions, but it was obvious that he really didn't want to know much about what had happened. I did not know how to prepare him for the insight that I felt would be a major step forward in his treatment. I was not experienced and knowledgeable enough at the time to use subtle "desensitizing" techniques to help Michael deal with the problem. [See page 131.]

At the end of the fifth session, he again let me know that he had no recall of what had happened. I told him about the spelling bee, his grandma and the eating for comfort and for fat protection. He didn't believe me. We discussed it some more. Then he panicked and ran from the office. Michael never came back and I never heard from him again.

I really blew that one. This incident is a good example of how not to help a patient confront reality. I was insensitive to Michael's needs and fears. I hadn't as yet even thought about such a thing as a craniosacral system. I was in the business of "fixing" people. I sure fixed Michael. I do thank him, if he is out there somewhere, because I have never forgotten the lesson he gave me. This lesson gains meaning with each year that passes in my life as a therapeutic facilitator. I now appreciate much more fully the work it may take to move from an unready to a ready conscious awareness.

Now let's consider another educational experience that a patient was kind enough to give me. This second example describes what can happen when the timing is right and conscious awareness is ready for a major piece of insight and self-awareness.

Reta was thirty-eight years old when she came to see me. The year was 1966. I was still pondering what had happened to Michael. He seemed to have disappeared. I had vowed never to be insensitive and overly forceful about reality confrontation again. Reta was the mother of four children, all still in school. She was the wife of an engineer who sometimes worked and sometimes didn't. She was the very valued, efficient and underpaid executive secretary of a local bank president.

Reta was referred to me because she had uncontrollable and unremitting pain in her head, neck, upper body, shoulders, arms, and hands. She also had episodically severe, but less frequent, low back and right sciatic pain. She was referred by an orthopedic surgeon who had operated on her three times already and couldn't find anything else to cut on. I had developed somewhat of a reputation as a pain controller who used hypnosis, trigger injection, manipulation, and whatever else was available. I also did a pretty fair brand of general medicine and minor surgery. Reta was probably a nuisance to the orthopedist by now, as well as a reminder that he had failed. He knew I would take the night calls because I was young and eager and rather taken with myself.

Reta had been surgically cut up and generally punished by life. She had her varicose veins surgically removed. She had a hysterectomy after her fourth obstetrical delivery. All four children were delivered vaginally with wide episiotomies. She then underwent a repair of the perineum and a bladder suspension (both done before the hysterectomy). Next she had her gallbladder removed. This referring orthopedic surgeon removed discs from between the third and fourth as well as the fourth and fifth lumbar vertebrae on two separate occasions. After this, he unsuccessfully attempted nerve-root decompression in the lower cervical region.

In addition to all this, her children were very demanding of her time and energy. They offered very little respect. Her husband abused her physically on occasion; he abused her psychoemotionally all the time. And her boss always asked for a little more than she could do.

Today this history would tell me of a need for self-punishment. Back then I just felt sorry for her. I simply listened to her story, examined her body, felt a lot of compassion, and vowed aloud that we would get to the bottom of this problem. Reta and I made a pact that we would both give it our best and go wherever the trail led us. This was very unprofessional behavior, even in those days.

I began to see Reta twice weekly. I started with trigger injection and manipulation. The first treatment produced relief for a few days. When the pain came back, it had changed its distribution somewhat and was a little worse in severity. To make a long story short, about ten sessions using trigger injection and manipulation got us nowhere. I recall the last trigger-injection session we had. The pain kept moving from one place to another around her upper back, thorax, neck, shoulders, arms and hands as I injected and manipulated. It was as though the pain was running away from my trigger injections. That night I injected eighteen triggers. This was a record for me, but we were determined to win.

Needless to say, we did not win with that approach. Reta's pain got much worse after that session. Hit by the sledgehammer of failure, I realized that trigger injections were not the way to fly. I thought

I had better think a little about what to do next. Meanwhile, Reta was unable to sleep because of her pain. I suggested she try to learn some self-hypnosis so that she could at least lessen the pain and get some sleep.

After a few sessions in which I attempted to teach her how to hypnotize herself to sleep, she spontaneously went into a deep trance. (This would suggest to me today that her nonconscious had checked me out and decided that I wasn't the best but was at least sincere and better than nothing.) I was suddenly inspired to search for the cause of the pain using hypnoregression. Almost immediately Reta regressed to memories beginning at age five and going down to when she was one year old. She lost her ability to converse as she got younger and younger and preverbal in her development. I suggested that her right hand would be able to write the answers to my questions as an adult, no matter how young she was during her experience. Lo and behold, she could do it. At age one she indicated that the reason for her pain had already been put into place. She simply wrote this information down for me on a stenographer's notepad.

I asked her to go back to the time when the reason for the pain was implanted. This was a tedious process because she could not talk intelligibly to me, so she had to write everything out. I didn't know at the time that I could have a part of her go up to the ceiling and be a "witness" to describe the scene to me. After many questions and a lot of slowly written answers (people write rather slowly under these circumstances), Reta regressed to age two days. She had been born at home and was lying in a cradle. Her mother and maternal grandmother were there. Her grandmother was admonishing her mother for having another baby at her age. The mother was forty-two, and Reta was the youngest of eight children. Grandma said that Reta should never have been born. It was too hard on the mother. Grandma also said that Reta would never be healthy.

The imposition of guilt and hopelessness brought upon Reta by this conversation was phenomenal. I shall never forget what Reta wrote when I asked her how she felt about this scene: "If I had to be born, if I have to live, at least I can be weak, sick, and hurt all my life."

When Reta came out of her regressed state, I very gently asked her if she could read what was written on the paper. She could not. She asked if I could read it, and I pretended I could not. She accepted my explanation without question because she wanted to believe me.

Three days later we repeated the same regression to the cradle, and she listened to her grandmother talking to her mother. She wrote me the same statement about how she felt. This time, I was a little wiser. I told her that the pregnancy had not been instigated by her. I told her that all had gone well. Her mother had survived the delivery without difficulty. I told her that her grandmother probably meant well but that her observations were not correct.

I wasn't sure I'd gotten through to Reta because she was still the two-day-old infant when I delivered my speech. I again let her know as she returned to the here and now that she did not need to comprehend anything she was not ready for. I was painstakingly careful about imparting the message to her. (I remembered Michael very clearly.) She could not read her handwritten message.

Four days later Reta came in again. Trance was quickly induced. I asked her to go to the experience that had convinced her she could not be without pain. She went straight to the same cradle scene. She heard her grandmother's words to her mother for the third time. I delivered my lecture again about the pregnancy not being Reta's responsibility. I then intuitively brought her back to adulthood while she was still in deep trance, and we discussed the situation.

Reta agreed that it was not valid that she should spend her life in pain because of her grandmother's emotional words to her mother. We also agreed that she would be able to handle the insight after she came out of trance. I brought Reta back to her usual state of conscious awareness. She was able to read her notes. (There were three sets of them by now.) She simply asked whether she could have done all of this to herself. I replied that it seemed reasonable.

Strange as it seems, that was the end of Reta's pain. She divorced her husband. She quit her job and started her own real estate company in partnership with a man who eventually became her husband.

Reta was an excellent teacher for me. I am forever grateful to her. In retrospect, Reta's case suggests that our nonconsciouses were definitely connected, even though I was not aware of it at the time. Why do I say this? There are several clues. Her pain got worse when I was doing the trigger injections. We made a pact to follow through to successful completion no matter what; I never did things like that. Intuitively I used hypnosis for sleep and pain control; Reta took it to hypnoregression. I was in way over my head trying to work with a two-day-old infant at that point in my career. I had no idea what to do, but looking back it feels like Reta's nonconscious told mine what to do. I then just followed my intuition without much forethought or question. Looks like a setup to me.

If I had gone easier with Michael or changed my timing, he might have come to grips with the cause of his obesity. As it was, I did him no favor. I only pray that he connected with his nonconscious at a later date and was able to handle what came up. With Reta, I listened more carefully—although I wasn't aware that I was listening. It worked out wonderfully well. Timing and sensitivity are critical. That which is unacceptable one moment might work fine an hour later.

One other point about timing that bears repeating: The therapeutic facilitator should always get the client to make the discoveries, no matter how much time it takes to get to them. As the facilitator, I must not just blurt out what is abundantly clear about the situation, but rather help patients make the discovery. I can make them thirsty and show them the water, but they have to do their own drinking.

A Case of Resistance

I worked with a young chiropractor who had gone into the profession largely because he had chronic, unrelenting low back and left leg pain. He had received all the adjustments he could handle, but the symptoms continued. I helped him develop his concept of an Inner Physician who was wise and knew all about his health and body.

We then developed a persona for this Inner Physician by requesting that he please come forward and get acquainted with us. We really wanted to talk with him because we needed his help. The Inner Physician presented himself as a wise man who gave out a kindly feeling. He said he understood the back and leg pain as well as its reason for existence. After much dialogue and rapport development, the Inner Physician agreed to show us the reason for the pain.

With some difficulty the patient re-experienced standing next to the bed as his older brother died of leukemia at home. The patient was three years old at the time. After strengthening the communication between nonconscious and conscious awareness, he could hear his aunt tell his mother, right after his brother took his last breath, that at least his brother wouldn't have any more pain. The patient's three-year-old mind interpreted this to mean that if you had pain you lived, and if you didn't have pain you died.

The nonconscious part of this patient made the interpretation that pain was a vital part of life; it therefore took on the job of making him hurt every day. It wasn't a pleasant task, but it seemed necessary. All we had to do was convince this part of the patient's nonconscious that life would go on and would be of better quality if the pain stopped. The pain did stop once he came to this realization, and it has not recurred since.

Desensitizing Techniques

While most of the desensitizing techniques have been introduced previously in this chapter, I would like to use this section to bring them all together.

By "desensitizing" I do not mean becoming numb or insensitive. Essentially, desensitization refers to the process of becoming better and better acquainted with a fearsome and powerful situation to the point that you are less susceptible to its emotional consequences. We use it in many aspects of practice.

A good example of desensitization is the ordinary process of "getting used to" cold water. We put our toe in the cold water first, then the foot, then both feet. Next we go in up to the knees and the thighs.

There is usually a longer wait before we get in up to the waist, but, once our lower region is acclimated, many of us will then dive into the water. Others will go in inch by inch until they are swimming. This is desensitization. Most of us have done it. Some people do not desensitize and don't go into the water all the way. There is also a macho group that will dive into anything. You usually hear a lot of yelling and screaming when it is done this way. I suppose this is rapid desensitization.

A patient I had been working with off and on for more than three years arrived one day in a state of near panic. Two days earlier she had been hit with a sudden onset of diarrhea followed by nausea and a little vomiting. Her world then began to spin incredibly. It was true vertigo that she described. Every time she changed her head position the world took off spinning. The nausea continued but the diarrhea never returned.

My tentative diagnosis was Meniere's disease, an inflammation of the semicircular canals in the inner ear that causes vertigo whenever the victim moves his or her head.

I asked the patient to lie down on the table. She said she could not. She said she had slept in a chair since her symptoms began.

I used the desensitizing principle to get her to lie down. I had her sit with her feet on the table and my hands on her head. I then had her lean back a few degrees—changing her head's orientation to gravity—until she began to get a little dizzy. We waited until the dizziness cleared. I kept my hands on her head. When her disequilibrium calmed down, as I supported her with my hands, I had her recline a little further until she wanted to stop again because of the return of the dizziness. We waited until her sense of equilibrium normalized. We then went a little further toward the supine position until she again had to stop. Five or six repetitions of the stop-wait-go process brought us to the supine position where I could effectively work on her cranium. I taught her how to do her own gentle ear pull, because the temporal bones are usually the chief offender in vertigo and Meniere's disease as far as the symptoms are concerned.

This is an example of a process of desensitizing. Each time we moved her head in relation to the gravitational orientation of the earth, we went slowly and gently. As we did, the equilibrium system became more and more accommodative of the movement. We went only as far as she would allow, then we stopped and waited until her inner ear adjusted. Had we gone too far or moved quickly and forcibly, the ensuing panic, both psychoemotionally and physiologically, would have put us right back at square one. We would have needed to overcome the resistance resulting from the bad experience before we could move on.

I explained what was happening physiologically as I worked with her, and by the end of the session she went from a supine to a sitting position without assistance. She felt some vertigo, but she calmly waited for the adjustment of her equilibrium to occur. She then stood, went over to the chair, sat down and waited for the vertigo to disappear. She had some very mild "spinny" feelings as she bent forward and put on her shoes, but she chose not to wait for it to clear because she knew it would come back for a short time after she sat straight up. It did and she waited a moment. She then stood, smiled, said thank you and was on her way.

She was desensitized. She had become familiar with the physiological dysfunction and she accepted it. She knew what it would do and when. She could now deal with her symptoms without the incapacitating panic and fear that had taken charge of her.

Desensitizing the client for therapeutic imaging and dialogue is essentially the same in principle as these examples. We also desensitize when we're restoring joint motion. We gradually increase the joint's tolerance to passive range of motion using many repetitions; we may then add active range of motion using lots of encouragement and assurance.

When we have clients who are nonconsciously confronting a very powerful and fearsome experience, we have to try to take the power away from the experience. We try to desensitize by familiarizing them with the experience. We let them know that when the event happened, it was immediately locked away in a strongbox by the nonconscious protector. The protector keeps it there because it is too horrible to look at. There is a fee, however, for the strongbox and for the non-conscious protector's services to guard it each month. These fees might take the form of nightmares every night, headaches every day, fear of strangers, acrophobia, chronic anger, mortal fear, pain anywhere in the body, or anything else you might dream of. There seems to be no limit to what can be self-imposed by the nonconscious.

How do we go about pulling the teeth out of such an experience? We must help the client put it in a different perspective so that it is less fearsome. To do this, we usually must examine the experience in detail. Let's take an example. The following case is one of the most fearsome and emotionally charged I have ever encountered.

A female patient about fifty years of age came in with unrelenting headaches. They were incapacitating for days at a time. The headaches had first begun when she was in her late teens. At that point they were controllable with pain medications. When she was about thirty years of age, the medication didn't work anymore. She went into psychotherapy and had been in it for about twenty years when she came to us for evaluation.

She went into SER on the first visit. It seemed that the headaches were a symptom under the control of a nonconscious part of her that was insisting on attention. The message was that she was sane; she must face the truth; and she must trust her memories and not the denials of her parents. Memories of what? We couldn't approach the material directly.

I developed a good speaking rapport and friendship with her headaches. The headaches then became the responsibility of an angel named Sam. Sam and I became quite close. We could dialogue without the patient being consciously aware of our conversation. I finally convinced Sam to share with me what it was that was locked away in the patient's strongbox and was so well protected.

Sam told me that childhood sexual abuse had begun when she

was less than a year old and had continued until the age of nine. The abuse included the mother, the father, and a string of deranged and perverted nannies.

Sam said the patient could probably handle knowledge of this material, although she had so far denied that it happened. There was one incident Sam felt was important for her to accept as fact. The patient was four years old. The mother and father were trying to perform a sex act her, but it was proving unsuccessful—her vagina was too small. Her mother finally took scissors and cut the tissues of her daughter's vagina to enlarge the orifice. Later, the mother got a little worried that a doctor seeing the girl's wounds might get suspicious. The story was therefore invented that she had fallen on an old swing-set pipe that was protruding from the ground in their backyard.

Now the mother and father began to brainwash the child. They convinced her that none of it was real, it was all her fantasy. They told her she was insane and would have to be put in an asylum if she told anyone of her fantasies. As long as she didn't tell anyone, though, they would keep the secret of her insanity and she could live at home. The parents felt secure in their secret and the sexual abuse continued for another four or five years.

Sam gave the girl headaches so that she would get attention and hopefully discover that she was sane, that these memories were real, and that it was her parents who were sick, not she.

How do you begin desensitizing something like this? I first had to let go of my repulsion. Then I began to investigate whether there were other parts of her nonconsciousness I could connect with. It turned out there were several who were eager to talk. There was, of course, the little girl. Along with her was an entity I will call "the protector," another named "Duke," and several other little girls of various ages. The first little girl tearfully described in more detail the events that Sam had previously told me about. I realized that this gradual unveiling of the story was part of the desensitization process, even though the patient was not yet consciously aware of our discussions.

Sam had accomplished the first step toward desensitization. The little girl herself then went further. In fact, she went through the experiences with me on several occasions, each time in more detail than the time before and with less fear. I helped her to realize that it was okay to come out of hiding, that her parents were mentally ill, and that she would not go to the asylum for telling what had happened. I also put her under the loving care of Sam the angel.

I next went to the "protector" and tried to convince him that the adult patient could perhaps handle the truth about her childhood in small doses. The protector was definitely the protector; he was very cautious. He held the key to the strongbox where the horrible memories were locked away. He softened a little but would not yet let any of these experiences come to conscious awareness. I worked with the protector some at each session. I made sure he was aware of the patient's progress toward truth.

Next I met "Duke." He was the angry, aggressive one. By description he reminded me of the Fonz (Henry Winkler) on the television show "Happy Days." Duke was tough and wanted to avenge the abuse, but he was not tough enough to go after Mother or Father. He did kick the nannies on occasion. Once, when a nanny was coming to get the girl ready for Mother and Father, Duke had the girl hide scissors under the mattress. As Nanny pinned her down, Duke reached around the mattress, grabbed the scissors and stabbed Nanny in the thigh. The woman ran out of the room screaming and resigned her position that night. The incident was denied by the mother and father. They said it was a dream. (Is it any wonder this patient was holding on to her sanity by a headache that was under the control of an angel named Sam?)

After this, the other little girls came forward, each with her own story of abuses. It really tested my ability to be non-judgmental and to believe in the significance detector, which told me that all this material was significant and, I believe, real.

After several sessions in which the patient began to get partial conscious awareness of some material as the protector let it out of his strongbox, I asked the patient to write a story about a little girl who was growing up in a home similar to her own. This was further desensitization. She wove bits and pieces of her life into her story. We then converted her story to a screenplay and imagined we were watching the movie together. More details of her childhood emerged as the movie progressed. I asked if she could play the lead in her movie. She finally agreed, and as she played the part she was further desensitized.

Finally, about the fourth time she played the part, she looked me right in the eye and said, "That little girl is me and that is what happened to me." This was a tough bit of reality to swallow. But at least she now knew what her headaches were about and that she wasn't crazy. Her headaches greatly improved after this, except when she allowed self-doubt to creep in. Once she felt sure again about what had happened in her life and trusted her sanity, the headaches went away. All this progress occurred in twenty-eight sessions over a period of four months.

By this time, the patient's father was dead. Her mother was still alive, though, so she decided to pay her a visit. While they were together, the patient's contact with reality softened and her headaches came back with a vengeance. She couldn't believe her mother did all those horrible things to her. As her self-doubt increased, so did her headaches. As she retrieved confidence in the truth of her memories, however, she experienced only moderate headaches. This has become the standard when she is away from her mother.

The problem is not totally resolved. She still has times when she can't believe this really happened to her. Perhaps she needs time to digest her insights. Maybe then she will be able to work with them herself. Whatever the case, I believe she will require a great deal of help. But at least she has had a look at her life and can see her reflection in the mirror.

Acceptance and Forgiveness

Once suppressed experiences, memories, emotions, and the like, come into conscious awareness, there is often the issue of what to do about the wrong that someone has done to a client. Perhaps a drunk driver killed a loved one or injured the client. Maybe the client was swindled, raped, witnessed a murder, or was abused by a parent or sibling. It could even be that God is being blamed for dealing the client a bad hand in life.

In alternative psychotherapies and "New Age" work, it is common to work toward forgiveness of a fellow human being who has somehow hurt, damaged or offended one. It is also reasonably common to work toward accepting the trials and tribulations attributed to God.

I remember how angry I was with God when he allowed my father to die shortly after my thirteenth birthday. I couldn't imagine how a "loving God" could do that. Now I accept that it happened and can find a rational reason.

Acceptance is defined as the state of accepting or being accepted. Webster's Unabridged Dictionary says that to accept is to take or receive what is offered with a consenting mind; to understand. Forgiveness is defined in the same dictionary as the state of forgiving, or a pardon. To forgive is to give up resentment or the desire to punish; to stop being angry. Both of these words, and the acts or states of mind they represent, are often misunderstood.

Many people think of acceptance as hopeless resignation. This is not so. Acceptance means that you take what comes and see what you can do about it without exercising anger or feeling vengeful. If you believe in reincarnation, you will probably be able to accept what comes—be it pleasant or unpleasant—as part of a greater plan. Thus, you may consider that every adverse situation, every accident, disease, and loss is a lesson. These adversities are challenges to be used to stimulate new growth and evolution.

True forgiveness is accepting and non-judgmental; it penetrates all levels and parts of the nonconscious and is filled with love. It is not a "Well, I guess so" act with reservations attached. Forgiveness is a word we often use incorrectly. I hear "I forgive him" used repeatedly in a condescending way. To some people, the ability to forgive implies that the forgiver possesses superior power over the forgivee. In this setting, forgiveness contributes to a hierarchy of "good" and "bad." The forgiver pardons the one he feels has hurt him, much as a governor pardons a criminal.

I try to be very careful not to contribute to this somewhat trite and hierarchical situation. Therefore, I do not use the word "forgiveness" very often. I use it only when I feel sure it is used correctly, from one human peer to another, or from one spiritual being to another. I believe that all earthbound humans have flaws and weaknesses, otherwise we wouldn't be here. We also have strengths and talents.

When you have been wronged by another, you have encountered one of that person's flaws or weaknesses. This may have been scripted before either of you was born, or it may have just happened that you were there when the weakness or flaw came out as an act of violence, robbery, deception, or the like. I try to remember that I, too, have weaknesses and flaws, and but for the grace of God the situation could be the other way around. What people frequently discover later is that it was the other way around at another time. Therefore, we should accept each other's imperfections.

Forgiveness is wonderful, but I find it important not to let the self-righteous patient use it to continue or create a "holier than thou" attitude. This happens a lot, and it simply creates further problems. Here is a dramatic example of how therapists who agree with the self-righteous attitude of a client can impede the therapeutic process.

The patient was a forty-year-old woman who began working with me to alleviate a severe problem with the joint connecting her lower jaw to her cranium (temporomandibular joint syndrome). She was in mouth splints and had been in braces.

SomatoEmotional Release began during the very first session. It became clear right away that as a child she had been sexually involved with her father. She later admitted that she had been in psychotherapy and counseling off and on for many years to get past the damage her father had done. She felt very angry, self-righteous and defiled. Her therapists through the years had supported the wrongness of her father's deeds.

After the first SomatoEmotional Release, I instinctively knew there was more to the sexual relationship with her father than she had uncovered during her years of therapy. I knew this because the issue was at the top of her nonconscious agenda. At subsequent sessions we used Therapeutic Imagery and Dialogue with SomatoEmotional Release to go detail by detail through her encounters.

What we got in touch with that the other therapists had missed was that she enjoyed the sex with her father. She was astonished at the enjoyment she felt, which included a sense of power over her authoritarian father while it was happening.

Her therapists had naturally placed her in the role of victim. They told her how badly she had been treated by her father and that he was a scoundrel. By making the father the abuser and her the victim, however, they did not allow room for her to remember the pleasure and sense of power that she felt. In this case, the therapeutic approach fostered powerful guilt because her nonconscious knew of her pleasure. The guilt then suppressed the pleasant memories and kept her in an emotionally destructive mode.

The result of all this inner turmoil? The temporomandibular joint syndrome that brought her to me in the first place. As she discovered that the things her father did to her were wrong in the eyes of society and her therapists, she was less and less able to open her mouth widely. The constant contraction of the jaw muscles created some inflammation of the joints. Once she confronted all the aspects of her experiences and let go of the guilt, the jaws relaxed and she healed wonderfully well.

Resolution and Application in Everyday Life

Once a person goes through all this catharsis and re-experiencing and gaining of insight, what does he or she do with it? How does it change that person's life?

I believe that the opening of communication lines between a patient's conscious awareness and the various regions of the nonconscious is the most important thing that can happen, so I generally develop a program to help keep them open.

I have the patient set up a time every day when the various characters who have come forward from the nonconscious meet with the patient's conscious awareness. This should be a pleasant meeting. It is very effective right upon awakening, before getting out of bed.

I help to set up an internal system of signals that are to be given the patient if he or she begins to neglect the meetings. I frequently suggest as a reminder the return of a familiar symptom that the patient consciously recognizes as controlled by the nonconscious. This could be an abdominal cramp, a stomach pain, a jab of sciatic pain, or anything that is mutually agreeable to the nonconscious and the conscious. This works really well and has about the same potency as a post-hypnotic suggestion.

Acceptance of what happened is important. Now that the experience is over, it's time to extract the lessons from it that are needed and move forward. It's time to get on with life and growth and healing. There is no place for self-pity, remorse, anger, resentment or revenge. I keep working with my patients until they either let it all go or refuse to do so. If they refuse, I try to help them see the cost of the destructive feelings they harbor.

Self-realization will usually change patients' lives. I used to think that I had to help them change. Now I just watch what happens. I trust the process. I don't go back and worry or fret. I don't try to redo it. I therapeutically facilitate the enhancement of self-awareness and knowledge. The enhanced self-awareness makes my patients better able to deal with what happens in the future. They are more independent. They don't need me. How does that feel? It feels good.

Chapter Five

The Fruits of Openness

Many people follow great teachers who facilitate their education and growth. My teachers are present, but they seem less tangible than most. They have given me examples to follow and have cast me into situations to learn from. The most important lesson they seem to offer out of all this is to be open and to observe.

For the rest of this book, I would like to share some aspects of my personal journey as a therapeutic facilitator, along with how I have been brought into the awareness of several extraordinary areas of reality— realities I had no idea I would find when I began my practice. I say that I have been brought to them because I do not believe I could have come to them on my own.

My Introduction to Acupuncture

In 1967 we opened two free clinics in Florida: one in St. Petersburg and the other in Clearwater. We treated a variety of people in need, including the poor, derelicts, young people in need of birth control and sex counseling, and a whole crop of drug abusers and addicts.

Butch Anderson, who was one of our clinic directors, had gone to San Francisco for a seminar for free-clinic directors. He returned with a small manual for pain control. It was originally written as a field manual for the barefoot doctors of North Korea. It had been translated into English long before Nixon went to China, so acupuncture was not yet a popular topic of conversation in this country. Butch showed me this little manual and I shrugged it off. Then he hit me in the ego department. "John, you're supposed to be open-minded. Why won't you try this? If it works we could save a lot on medicine in the clinics."

So I read the booklet. It was about forty pages with illustrations. The last chapter showed nine points to needle that, the text claimed, would relieve pain anywhere in the body. When inserted, the needles were supposed to be comparable in analgesic potency to a quarter grain of morphine. The advantage of the needles was that they would not interfere with mental functioning as morphine did. They had been used to ease the pain of wounded soldiers who needed to be transported to medical facilities and still have their wits about them.

I was pretty skeptical, but Butch kept after me until I finally agreed to try it on three very difficult pain patients. One was a young man with acute rheumatoid arthritis. The second was a man in his sixties who was in constant and severe pain from terminal bone cancer that had spread to the lumbar spine from the prostate gland. The third was an alcoholic woman in her late fifties with chronic pain in her liver and biliary duct system. She had bile in her urine almost constantly. An examination of this system during surgery to remove her gallbladder had revealed no other problems that would cause this condition. I therefore felt that the contamination of bile in the urine was due to residual liver disease from long years of alcohol abuse. We had no answer for her continuous acute pain.

I thought these three patients would be an effective challenge to the nine magic needle placements described in the little booklet. If the pain was relieved, acupuncture would have my attention. If it was not relieved, Butch had agreed to get off my back.

I used 25-gauge disposable hypodermic needles. With the book in one hand and a needle in the other, I put nine needles in each of these three patients. Each needle went in about half an inch. I'm sure I must have inspired a lot of confidence as I read the book, mumbled under my breath, and jabbed the needles into the three patients. The plan was to leave the needles in place for about thirty minutes. I know you are just dying to know where the needles were placed. The points were: Large Intestine 4, both sides; Stomach 36, both sides; Gallbladder 36, both sides; Pericardium 4, both sides; and Governing Vessel 16.

Within ten minutes the patient with rheumatoid arthritis said his pain was all gone. He remained in remission for two days, then the pain returned. He would not come in for another treatment. My suspicion was that being pain-free scared the heck out of him—as did my obvious amateur status as an acupuncturist.

The cancer patient got about seventy-five percent relief from pain within thirty minutes. I showed his wife, a licensed practical nurse, where and how to insert the needles. I marked the points with a skin pencil. She needled him twice a day as he needed it, always using the same points and the 25-gauge disposable needles. He needed no narcotics after this. He did very well with the needles as his pain control method until he died about two months later.

The third patient was the most remarkable. She was pain-free by the time I got the last needle in place, and she remained that way for twenty-four hours. What is even more remarkable is that the color of her urine changed from a bile-stained greenish-yellow to a normal color for about two days. She came in for follow-up treatments about three times a week.

After some experimentation I finally found that, in her case, I could insert one needle just below the rib cage on the right side of her body and achieve pain relief for a few hours. (I didn't know anything about meridians at that time.) This was easier than using all nine needles. I did the one-needle treatment a few times. I then decided to leave this one needle in place with antibiotic cream on the puncture site and a bandage over it for three days, rather than do one needle for fifteen to thirty minutes two or three times a week. The urine remained clear of bile while the needle was in place, but the bile returned about eight or nine hours after I took the needle out.

I needed to find something besides a needle to stimulate this area. The needle did the job systemically, but it was too irritating. I put a rather heavy-gauge silk suture through this point and tied a little chain on it—the type found on old-fashioned drain plugs. I put antibiotic cream over the suture, covered it with a large bandage, and let the chain hang down. I told her that whenever she had the pain she should pull the chain intermittently until the pain stopped. I was just guessing. I asked her to change the bandage every day, clean the area with peroxide, and apply fresh antibiotic cream.

After about two weeks of chain pulling, the time between pulls became longer and longer. Finally, the pain didn't return and the urine stayed clear. She had completely recovered.

That patient taught me a lot about open-mindedness, about not being afraid to try what seems to make sense. She also reminded me that in modern medicine we are really only scratching the surface. She and I stayed in touch for at least five years after her remarkable recovery. Her liver and bile duct problems did not surface again clinically during that time. To my knowledge, she never drank alcohol again. She was certainly a great teacher.

Acupuncture Becomes a Regular Part of My Practice

I had a few more really eye-opening and mind-expanding experiences with acupuncture in the late sixties. After that first experience with pain alleviation, I was moved to do some study of the acupuncture system. I found an Oriental bookstore catalogue through the San Francisco-based Free Clinic Association. A British internist, Felix Mann, had authored four books on the subject. I felt that any British internal medicine specialist who could write four books on the subject must be pretty good, so I sent for all four of them.

I didn't have the books more than a week when a woman came in with acute shingles (herpes zoster) on her right side. She was twenty-five years old and almost hysterical from the pain—probably due in some part to the fact that she was prone to hysteria. She came to see me after her family doctor had injected cortisone and it hadn't helped. A friend told her that I was good with difficult problems. I looked at the rash and knew that it hurt a lot. I tried to palpate the rib angles and

Acupuncture

The organs: Organs in acupuncture are not exactly the same as they are in our Western physiology. The organs include not only the physical heart, lungs, kidneys and so forth, but the type of energy associated with them and the meridians or channels along which that energy flows—either from the organ, through the body, to the surface where the meridian terminates at the ends of the fingers or toes; or from the terminating points towards the organ. The energy (chi) of the organs can be accessed at specific points along the meridians by means such as inserting needles (acupuncture), applying manual pressure (acupressure), or burning special substances over the points (moxibustion).

The organs along with their meridians and chi are characterized as yin or yang. Health in general is identified with a proper yin/yang balance, and diagnosis and treatment attempt to restore yin/yang imbalances.

The meridians are named according to the organ systems with which they are associated. The points along the meridians are numbered in sequence, in accordance with the direction along the meridians that the chi energy is said to flow. Thus, "Liver 3" is the third point along the liver meridian.

Traditional Chinese medicine associates the organs with a theory of five elements and correlates the functioning of the organs with the seasons. The organs are also associated with specific emotional qualities. Deficiencies or excesses in the energy of a given organ may express themselves as imbalances in the emotional life of the patient. Treatment by acupuncture essentially integrates physical symptoms with emotional qualities.

vertebrae in the mid-thoracic area and she almost fainted.

Then it came. Eureka! Let's try acupuncture.

I had scanned Dr. Mann's books once. There was no index, so I started looking through the contents of one of them: *Acupuncture: Treatment of Many Diseases.* I found what I was looking for: "Intercostal Neuralgia" (nerve pain between the ribs). There was a list of acupuncture points to treat, but no explanation about how the treatment points had been selected.

I extended Dr. Mann the courtesy of trust and used the points indicated for the pain on her right side. I inserted the 25-gauge disposable hypodermic needles. Some insertion points bled and some didn't. Within minutes her pain subsided significantly and the redness of the rash blanched. She became totally pain-free and her hysteria subsided.

My treatment schedule was based on how she felt. She called me every day to report how things were going. I treated her five more times using the same acupuncture points. That was the end of the shingles. She was eternally grateful.

Within the next few months, I was bombarded with more than thirty cases of shingles. Acupuncture worked so well that I was propelled into the practice in the space of just a few short weeks.

There are three more acupuncture experiences that I must relate because they were so mind-expanding. First is the case of a forty-eight-year-old nurse who had suffered from a brain tumor. The tumor had been removed by the neurosurgeon at our hospital, but she developed acute facial pain after the surgery. The surgeon called to ask if I would try acupuncture on her. I agreed with the caveat that it would be exploratory.

Out came the by now famous and trusted manual of Felix Mann, M.D. I looked up facial pain and added a few of my own ideas about opening exit points to release the pain from the meridians that passed through those areas. (By then I had some smaller 27-gauge disposable needles to use.) The Bladder 1 acupuncture point is at about the same spot where the nose piece for old-fashioned eyeglasses rests. I put in all of the other needles and told her I'd be back in ten minutes to see how she was doing. I had a busy office and it was my practice to treat several patients at the same time.

When I came back to remove the needles, the needle in Bladder 1 on the painful right side had been drawn into the tissue up to its nub, and its point was aimed directly at the eyeball. Originally I had just barely penetrated the deep side of the skin with this needle and the point was aimed at the nose. (Incidentally, the Bladder 1 needle on the non-painful left side was still as I had placed it.) I asked if she had tampered with the needles. She said no, and I really had no reason to disbelieve her. I gently tried to retract the needle. It would not budge. I tapped, I twirled, I wiggled it. Nothing helped. I removed the other needles. Bladder 1 on the right showed no sign of loosening. I decided I would have to use brute force. It was like pulling a really tough weed. When it finally came out, there was tissue attached to the last half-centimeter of the needle. This accounted for the difficult removal.

I sent the needle to the pathology department at the hospital. The pathologist called to ask me what I was doing at my office. He reported that the needle had had a rather large quantity of fibrous connective and muscle tissue fused to it, as if by either heat or electricity. He used the analogy of meat being fused to a skewer after it has been cooked too long over an open pit. He said he had not seen anything like this before. I told him I hadn't either. There was no heat or electricity used in this treatment. In fact, I doubted that I had even touched the metal needle shaft because I always held only the plastic nub of the disposable needle to make the insertion.

This experience certainly made a statement about there being some kind of energy within the body that was not dependent upon external sources. I have not seen this happen since this first experience, but I certainly cannot dismiss this observation simply because I have not seen it twice. The patient's facial pain, it turned out, was due to a local infection. After it was opened and drained, she responded well to acupuncture treatment.

The next astonishment I experienced was a case of secondary heart failure that was not responding to traditional medical care. Harold was a big, robust, happy man in his late sixties. I had been his family doctor for a couple of years. Suddenly, for no reason I could discover, he began to suffer episodes of acute shortness of breath, irregular heartbeat, fluid retention, and the whole syndrome that we call cardiac asthma. He was hospitalized four times in three months. During his fourth hospitalization, I asked cardiology for help because

I was getting nowhere. Harold went home from that stay with digitalis to control his heart ventricles, quinidine to control the atria of his heart, six Lasix a day to get rid of his excess body fluid, prednisone to help keep his lungs clear, an inhaler to use when he got short of breath, and an oxygen tank, just in case.

He came to the office about three days after being discharged. He told me that if this was how he had to live, he would rather die. I didn't much blame him. He asked about "this here acupuncture" that he heard I was fooling around with. I told him I had no idea how to treat him with acupuncture. He said he trusted me and was sure I could figure out what to do. How could I refuse?

I had been fooling around with Chinese pulse diagnosis as described by Felix Mann. I had accepted that acupuncture needling worked, but diagnosis by pulse seemed preposterous to me. Nonetheless, Dr. Mann said it was reliable, so I examined Harold's pulses. Oddly enough, his heart and lung pulses seemed full and vital, but I couldn't find his kidney pulse. My surprise probably showed on my face. Harold encouraged me to "go for it," so I did.

I put needles in all the kidney stimulation points I could discover on Dr. Mann's chart. I did nothing else except tell Harold to come back in twenty-four hours and bring all of his urine with him in a clean gallon milk jug.

The next day at 2 P.M. Harold came in cussing and raising hell in a good-humored way that I hadn't seen him display in four or five months. He announced to those in the waiting room that he hadn't slept all night because he was up "pissin'." Harold had produced almost two gallons of urine during the night, and he had lost sixteen pounds according to our scales. He felt great.

I never had to treat Harold's kidneys by acupuncture or any other method again. Once was enough. His kidney pulses were palpable the next day. I weaned him from his medicine over about a week's time and we turned in his oxygen tank. He never had another problem with his heart, lungs or kidneys after that. He even had uneventful lumbar disc surgery in 1973. His heart did fine.

This was certainly another mind-expanding experience for me. I have trusted the pulses and my ability to use them ever since. In his previous hospital stays, Harold had showed no signs of kidney problems. It all seemed to be heart and lungs. The pulses contradicted the Western diagnosis.

I sure didn't know what to make of this. How could the position and pressure of a finger on the radial artery tell if a guy like Harold had heart, lung or kidney problems as his primary ailment? So much to learn. Thank you, Harold.

The next acupuncture experience that further expanded my mind and increased my humility came by way of Linda. Linda was a very attractive single woman in her mid-twenties. She was an upward-bound, successful professional in the legislative branch of state government.

Linda presented with a very acute case of genital herpes. The labia of the vagina were very red and terribly swollen. She could not bear to have anything touch this area of her body, including underwear. Her acute pain and distress prompted me to try steroid and local anesthetic injections into the lower sacral regions. I was trying to treat the triggers to the area. I did relevant osteopathic manipulation and provided her with a topical anesthetic spray, which I hoped would ease the pain and perhaps interrupt the segmental facilitation.

She was back in two days. She was no better. In fact, she was perhaps a little worse. I really didn't know what to do. Then it struck me: Let's try acupuncture. I again looked through Dr. Mann's table of contents in *Acupuncture: Treatment of Many Diseases*. This time I could find nothing relevant. Then I remembered that Dr. Mann stated in one of his other books that the Chinese view pain as "fire." I decided that I needed to let the fire out of the kidney and bladder meridians that controlled and/or passed through the painful areas.

I used the fire points to loosen or mobilize the pain on the meridians. I used the exit points to let the fire pain out of the meridian once it was mobilized. And I used the source points because my understanding was that they would act homeostatically, letting chi (energy) in or out depending on what was appropriate. I felt that letting out all that fire/pain energy might drain the meridian. I wasn't sure, though, so I used the source point. I figured I would let the acupuncture point decide what was appropriate, because I certainly didn't know what I was doing. I used the disposable hypodermic needles bilaterally in the fire, exit and source points of both the kidney and bladder meridians.

Within minutes of the needle insertion, Linda's pain began to subside. I had her positioned on the gynecology table with her feet and legs in stirrups so that I could observe the vaginal labia. The labial swelling began to reduce. I could touch the labia without Linda screaming in agony. Within thirty minutes the pain and swelling were at least eighty percent gone.

I treated Linda three more times on consecutive days. When we finished the third treatment, there were no more subjective symptoms, although I could still see a little minor swelling of the labia majora. I did follow-up pelvic exams and Pap smears every six months for about two years after this episode. There was no recurrence of the herpes during that time.

What next? Now you can let pain out of the body like turning on a faucet!

Your Whole Body Is on Your Ear!

I had accepted and used body acupuncture successfully. I had been astonished to see the diagnostic reliability of pulse diagnosis. Now I was presented with the ridiculous idea that the whole body is represented on the ear.

I had just read a book titled *Auriculotherapy* by French physician Paul F.M. Nogier, in which he described the homunculus on the ear. He explained that the ear cartilage represents the bones of the spine, the outer edge of the ear the spinal cord, and so forth.

In no way could I accept this—until I fell through an eighteen-foot scaffold one day while putting a roof on our house. I did a nice para-

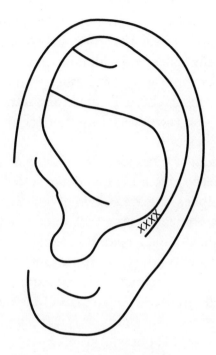

Illustration 5-1.
X's indicate area of treatment that relieved pain in lower cervical and upper thoracic spine. Treatment consisted of simply compressing the area quite firmly between my thumb on the back of the ear and my index fingernail on the front of the ear. Compression was held two to three minutes at a time and repeated frequently throughout the day in response to return of pain. Within four to five days, pain no longer returned.

trooper landing on the brick patio. As I rolled backward from my feet to my buttocks, the bundle of shingles that I'd had on my shoulder fell on my head. The shingles were followed very shortly by two pieces of the two-by-twelve board that had conveniently broken in order to let me fall through the scaffolding. I learned about time warp on the way down. It felt like it took several minutes to go from eighteen feet in the air to the brick patio.

The result of all this? My head was pounded down into my spine to about the third and fourth thoracic vertebrae. In retrospect, I realize that I had put a dandy energy cyst into my upper thoracic spine.

After the incident I had about fifty osteopathic manipulations from two or three of my colleagues with little or no relief. I had a constant pain in my upper spine and related muscles, the scapulae, the shoulders, and both arms. I felt like I wanted about five hundred pounds of traction to pull on those vertebrae to decompress them. No one seemed able to help me.

I thought about Nogier's ideas in *Auriculotherapy* as I drove to the hospital one afternoon to make my rounds. I took my left ear between my thumb and index finger. I started pressing on the cartilage in the areas where the cervical and upper thoracic vertebrae and soft tissue were represented. I found a place that really "hurt good" and pressed with my fingernail. As I did, my ear hurt more, but my whole upper-back and arm-shoulder pain syndrome started to ease up.

My pain syndrome was enough to motivate me to do this ear pressure at least four or five times a day. The syndrome continued to improve and nearly disappeared after about two weeks. I suppose I should thank the scaffolding company for sending me a defective plank. Or perhaps I could thank whomever arranged this scenario; it seems to be more than a coincidence.

Soon I was successfully using ear acupuncture on patients in conjunction with body acupuncture. I then started to inject minuscule drops of vitamin B12 into the addiction points of the ear in order to treat narcotics addicts. It worked beautifully to ease the withdrawal syndrome and reduce the desire for more drugs. This experience opened another world for me.

Opening to the Psychic

In the late sixties I was pretty sure that psychics, fortune-tellers, healers, and the like, were all a bunch of con artists. (I was perhaps a little bit open on this subject, but not much.) Around 1970, the real forces of the universe decided to run me through a series of experiences in order to open my mind to the reality of psychic phenomena. I was thirty-eight years old and was engaged at the time in a rather acute-care osteopathic medical and surgical practice: A lot of heart attacks, strokes and traumas from the beaches were my daily fare. I also had purchased a two-hundred-seat restaurant and lounge. (I should mention that I have been a jazz pianist since my youth. All jazz musicians want to have their own club someday. I managed to do it!)

One evening my bartender/manager, Gordon, came to me and said, "Doc, you need to get a replacement for me." I asked why. I thought Gordon was happy. As far as I knew we were good friends. Gordon said that he had just seen a psychic named Harriet in St. Petersburg. Harriet told him that within three months he would take a new job at a salary of $25,000 per year, plus have an expense account and a company Lincoln to drive. He would wear a suit and tie every day. I hid my disbelief to some extent but not very well, I'm sure. Gordon had not completed high school. He was bright and experienced in the bar business, but what did an old psychic lady living in St. Petersburg know about how the world really worked? (Boy, would I live to eat my words.) I promptly forgot the incident.

About a month later Gordon gave me two weeks' notice. He had been offered a job by two land developers who had come by the club for a drink. They liked his style and hired him right out from under me. He was to meet prospective real estate customers at the airport, show them the land development project, and deliver them to the office for the sales pitch. For this work he would receive a $25,000 annual salary, an expense account, and a Lincoln in which he was to chauffeur the potential buyers; plus, he was to wear a suit and tie every day.

This was some coincidence! I thought to myself, it just goes to show how psychics like Harriet get their reputation. Every once in awhile they are right. I supposed that if you guessed enough you had to hit it right once in a while. What a fine rationalization!

Within a few months, my wife and office nurse announced they were going together to see Harriet for a "reading." When my wife entered her reading room, Harriet exclaimed, "Oh, you poor dear, your husband is in the hospital." Then Harriet calmed down and said, "It's okay, he's a doctor; he's seeing his patients." This was true.

That afternoon, I left the hospital to pick up our son at the YMCA, where I had dropped him off earlier to go swimming. Arriving fifteen minutes ahead of schedule, at 3:45 P.M., I went to the bowling alley next door to wait. My stomach was a little upset, so I ordered a glass of beer, which I really didn't want.

My wife, who was with Harriet at the time, told me that Harriet interrupted the reading at 3:50 P.M. to tell her how foolish I was to drink a glass of beer when I really didn't want it. I was sure at that point that Harriet was working some sort of scam and was having me followed. How the instant communication occurred between the person tailing me and Harriet I didn't know, but I sure didn't believe that some old psychic could know that I drank a glass of beer I didn't want at ten minutes to 4. (Come to think of it, how would the tail know I didn't want it? But I didn't think of that at the time.) In retrospect, I can certainly see how far we reach to explain something logically that we don't want to believe.

The events with Gordon and my wife piqued my curiosity to the point that I decided to see Harriet myself. When I called to make an appointment, a pleasant voice answered, "Hello, my dear." Could this be the mysterious psychic? She sounded more like Betty Crocker or Mrs. Olsen. I asked for a consultation for the following Monday morning if that was possible. Harriet said that would be fine, and we set the appointment for 11 A.M. on Monday. I asked if she wanted my name. She said, "No, I don't need a name. I know you'll be here." I asked how she knew that. She said that knowing such things was what she did.

At 11 A.M. on Monday I arrived at the back steps of a rather old, but pleasant and cheery, frame house with lots of flowers in the yard. I was in paint-stained hobby jeans, moccasins, and a tee shirt. I had driven my old Austin Healy Sprite. I was sure that no one would ever guess I was a doctor. I stood at the top of three wooden steps and rapped on the screen door. Looking through the screen I saw a very

pleasant kitchen done predominantly in bright yellow. A plump, cheru-
bic, white-haired, rosy-cheeked grandmotherly kind of person came
to the door. I said, "Good morning, I have an appointment at 11 A.M.
Is Harriet here?"

The woman said, "Good morning, my dear. I've been waiting for
you. You're the osteopath. I have a sore shoulder and you can fix it."
I could not come up with a logical explanation for how she knew I
was an osteopath. I hadn't even given a first name when I made the
appointment. I was temporarily disarmed. It would get worse very
quickly.

Harriet invited me in and asked if I would fix her shoulder before
our reading. She said there was plenty of time. She had planned lunch
for both of us after the consultation was over. She sat on a kitchen
chair and I stood behind her, somewhat at a loss what to do. I began
to work on her neck and upper back.

She said very quickly, "Oh no, you needn't bother with all that; just
put your hands on my shoulders." I didn't question or object, I just
cupped one hand over each shoulder. My left hand began to get warm.

Harriet said, "Oh you poor dear, you don't have quite enough
energy. Blue Belle, come and help him." Within a second—I swear to
you—the pantry door flew open. Very quickly my hand became
uncomfortably hot. Harriet's shoulder was better right away. There
weren't any electronic bugging devices or private detectives that could
do this. My belief system did an about-face. She had convinced me.

Harriet and I became rather good friends after that first consultation. I went to see her on Mondays for several consecutive weeks. We
treated each other and consulted and had lunch together. Harriet
answered any questions I asked.

During our first session she totally astonished me. She became a
different old lady and spoke to me in German, which I could not
understand. When she reverted back to herself, she told me that the
German lady was Mary Wahl and she wanted me to keep my feet dry
and warm where I was going. (Mary Wahl was my paternal grandmother, who had died when I was three years old. Wahl was her

maiden name.) What did this advice mean? I didn't know at the time that I would be moving to Michigan in 1975, after eleven years living in Florida.

Harriet also told me not to worry about the book; it would be finished and be a big success. (I hadn't even thought of CranioSacral Therapy yet, let alone written a book about it.) In addition, she told me that two "doctors" were competing for my attention. One was a brown-skinned Polynesian acupuncturist and the other was a tall Caucasian man named Henry White.

The name Henry White jogged my memory. While I was a biochemistry fellow in Kirksville, Missouri, I was given an old library storage room for my office. I went through hundreds of dusty old books that were stored there. One of the old books was a notebook dated 1901 that contained the class notes of an osteopathic student named Henry White. I really enjoyed reading those notes. One day when I went to look for the notebook, it just wasn't there. I had always wondered where it went. I still don't know, but what a coincidence that Harriet would see a spirit guide named Henry White who wanted to direct me along a given path. (I don't know who the Polynesian acupuncturist was, but I guess he had the upper hand in guiding me at the time since I was doing about twenty acupuncture treatments a week.)

As we became friends, Harriet told me a few things that I'll share with you. She said that my education was one of the assignments she had to complete before she died. She told me that on a bad day her skills were merely telepathic and she could only tell clients what they were thinking, which was still enough to impress them satisfactorily. On a good day, however, she could connect with the spirit guides around a person. If the guides were nice she would let them use her body to communicate. If bad spirits came around, she just told them to "be gone," and they would leave because she wasn't afraid. She told me that life's scenarios are preconceived by the spirits before we are born. We can cooperate with the scenarios and have a relatively easy life, or we can be obstinate and contrary and have a difficult life.

It is really our individual choice.

Harriet said that a single soul can divide and be two or more incarnate humans in order to play out a scenario and learn a lesson. (This explains the population explosion to some extent.) Most souls don't really enjoy the earthly life; it is just something they have to do in order to advance.

During that first consultation Harriet had also predicted, quite accurately, that my family and I would move north into a house on a hill with water in the back, but the move wouldn't be permanent. We moved to Michigan in July 1975 and bought a large brick house on a hill with a marsh out back.

Harriet astonished me one day when she told me that she was diabetic and gave herself insulin injections. I inquired as to how many calories she ate per day and how many units of insulin she took. She said it was different every day. She pushed my "regular doctor" button with that statement. I delivered my lecture on balancing the number of calories and units of insulin with controlled exercise. She just said, "Oh my dear, that sounds so complicated. For about twenty-five years now I've been taking whatever dose of insulin Blue Belle tells me to take every morning." I conceded that Blue Belle knew more about diabetes management than I did. Harriet lived to her mid-eighties. I'm sure she finished her assignments and that the variable dosage of insulin had little or nothing to do with her demise.

Harriet truly changed my life.

The Discovery of CranioSacral Therapy

After acupuncture let me know how little I really knew about how bodies work, and Harriet let me know that psychic phenomena and psychics are real, I must have become properly open because along came Delbert. He is the man many of my students have heard me describe as the person back in 1971 who gave me my first and irrefutable personal look at the craniosacral system as a semiclosed hydraulic system. I told this story in more detail in my book, *Your Inner Physician and You.*

I received a call from Delbert's daughter, Sandy, asking me to please stop by and see her father that morning on the way to the hospital. I had been her family doctor for some time. In fact, I had delivered her son. I had never seen Delbert before. I did know that he was a retired coal miner from West Virginia and supposedly had some degree of black lung disease.

I arrived at Delbert's home around 9 A.M. I was greeted by Sandy and Delbert's wife, Geneva. Delbert was on the living room floor. The place smelled of whiskey. There was vomit on the floor with partially digested food and fresh blood in it. Delbert was only semiconscious and looked like "death warmed over," as my mother used to say. I was a little upset with Sandy because she hadn't mentioned to me that her father was an alcoholic, which was my immediate assessment. I checked Delbert's vital signs. His blood pressure was low and his heart rate rapid. Who could tell how long or how much he had been bleeding. If this was alcoholism, he was probably bleeding in the esophagus from varicose veins, which usually develop from increased back pressure from the liver. If that was the case, his life expectancy was really poor.

I decided to get him to the hospital by ambulance to avoid wasting time. I tried to get Sandy or Geneva to tell me that Delbert was an excessive user of alcohol, but both denied it. They wouldn't have had much motivation to lie to me now, so maybe something else was wrong. They said he drank some whiskey that morning to ease the pain in his stomach. Then he vomited the whiskey. That was when Sandy called me, and that was why the place reeked of booze. The ambulance arrived and we all left for the hospital.

The original diagnostic workup I did with Delbert revealed liver dysfunction along with cystic formation at multiple sites in both the liver and brain. This was not, however, the generalized liver disease associated with alcoholism. As expected, the lungs confirmed black lung disease of ancient origin. The stomach demonstrated some active ulceration. The esophagus did not show varicosities, so apparently the fresh blood I saw in the vomit was gastric in origin.

Now we had to discover the cause of the cysts and ulcer. Blood tests showed that Delbert was quite anemic, which was no real surprise. Through a liver biopsy and blood agglutination test, we were finally able to trace the probable cause to a systemic infection by a parasite named Echinococcus. Delbert responded well enough to conservative medical treatment, and I discharged him from the hospital after about three weeks.

Shortly after discharge he called me and said that the bottoms of his feet hurt so badly that he couldn't walk. I stopped by his home on the way to the hospital one morning. The soles of his feet were cracked, peeling and rather black in color. I had never seen or heard of anything like this in my young career. I asked around the staff at the hospital and got no helpful suggestions. The dermatologist I sent Delbert to was of no help either.

Then began the trek of referrals to medical centers—first to a medical center in Gainesville, Florida, then to Duke University in Durham, North Carolina, and finally to a facility for coal miners in West Virginia. The answers we got from those institutions related mostly to central nervous system problems, pulmonary disease, liver dysfunction (which was mild by now), and some constitutional inadequacy. There were no answers concerning the problem with his feet, and Delbert wasn't complaining about anything but his feet. After all of this, Sandy and Geneva prevailed upon me to hospitalize Delbert once more to see if I could find the answer. I was not optimistic.

A new neurosurgeon had just joined the staff. He had been in general practice for nine years before undertaking a general surgical residency in the United States and neurosurgical training in Japan. He had some new and different ideas—or at least they were new to me. I asked him to examine Delbert. He did and suggested there might be a problem in the cervical area of the meninges. In Japan he had seen this problem cause pathological responses elsewhere in the body. The problem with the skin of the feet might be due to some form of dystrophy.

He recommended a cervical myelogram. (This was prior to CT

scans, MRIs and ultrasound diagnostic techniques.) We had to put a radio opaque dye in the subdural space. Then we tilted the x-ray table head-down so that the dye, which was injected in the lumbar region and was heavier than cerebrospinal fluid, would get into the cervical area. There we saw it: an epidural (outside of the dura mater) calcification about a centimeter in diameter and perhaps one-fifth of a centimeter thick covering the midline in the mid-cervical region.

When the neurosurgeon suggested that the cervical plaque (the calcification) could be causing the foot problem, I was quiet and decided to go along with his ideas. After all, we had no other worthwhile leads to follow. We decided that we had better get that plaque of calcium out of there before it created further problems. I was a little surprised that a cervically located plaque on the outside of the dural membrane could cause the bottoms of the feet to become sore, turn black, and peel off. Yet I was also running out of the ability to be surprised after my experiences with acupuncture and my good friend Harriet. (I should have asked Harriet what was wrong with Delbert, but I didn't think of doing that until much later.) In any case, we scheduled the surgery to remove the calcified plaque.

In order to perform the surgery, Delbert was put in a sitting position, leaning forward, in an anesthesia chair. This position gave us good access to the back of his neck. We used a midline incision. We removed the posterior parts of the fourth cervical vertebra and opened a nice round operative field. Once the external surface of the dura mater was exposed, there was our calcified plaque staring us in the face. The neurosurgeon instructed me to hold the dural membrane very still with Allis clamps so that he could remove the plaque from the dural membrane without cutting or puncturing this tissue. Little did I know that this would be my first look at the craniosacral system.

As I rather unsuccessfully tried to hold this membrane still, I realized it was moving rhythmically centralward into the operative site and then peripheralward toward the outside of the body through the operative site. Neither the neurosurgeon nor the anesthesiologist had ever noticed anything like this before. Both were a little impatient with my questions because the idea of surgery is to get in, do your job, and get out. There is not much tolerance for wasting time. Despite their impatience, I managed to time this rhythmical activity at about eight cycles per minute. It was not in synchrony with the patient's breathing, which was visible from the breathing bag in the anesthesia machine. And it certainly was not synchronous with the heart action, which was visible on the cardiac monitor. It was a rhythm none of us in the operating room had ever witnessed.

I felt at the time that I was the only one who cared. I was puzzled a little as I watched the dural membrane moving in and out of the operative site, despite my efforts to hold it still. It seemed to me that about the only mechanism that could produce this effect would be a rhythmical rise and fall in fluid pressure on the other side of the membrane. This suggested to me that the dural membrane was involved in a hydraulic pumping system that I knew very little about.

It was this experience that started me on the path of clinical and basic scientific research which ultimately led to the development of CranioSacral Therapy, SomatoEmotional Release, and all the rest. Delbert and his Echinococcus really changed my life.

As for Delbert, his feet returned to normal within about two months of the surgery. Sadly, he died of lung cancer in 1981.

Cranial Osteopathy: One Major Step Along the Way

I was introduced to cranial osteopathy in my sophomore year at osteopathic college (late 1959/early 1960) by a visiting lecturer from The Cranial Academy. Very few of us took this lecture seriously because he talked about the rhythmical movement of skull bones, which most of us believed was nonsense. I thought no more about the matter—until the experience with Delbert.

Following Delbert's surgery, I continued to be mildly puzzled about the movement of the dural membrane I had witnessed. I did not make the connection right away, though, with the instruction I had received so many years previously.

Then one day a notice in the *Journal of the American Osteopathic Association* caught my eye. It was an invitation to a five-day course in cranial osteopathy. The claim was that participants would learn to feel the movement of skull bones and how to use that movement to treat various conditions related to impaired skull-bone motion. I decided to attend the course because it might be connected to what I had witnessed during Delbert's surgery.

A most impressive review of the anatomy of the skull and sacrum was presented, followed by an opportunity to experience the techniques the lecturers had just talked about. When Dr. Wales, my supervising instructor, put her hands on my head, my head began to feel like Jell-O. I could feel all sorts of movements inside it. Then she put her hand under my sacrum and the same thing happened: my pelvis seemed to turn to Jell-O. Both my skull and pelvis were rhythmically moving. By the time it was my turn to do the hands-on work, it was as though I had been feeling this motion for years. I still did not accept the ostepathic explanations of why this movement was present, but I certainly could not deny that I was feeling it.

I went back to my practice and used the cranial osteopathic techniques on the first three severe and chronic headache patients who came in asking for acupuncture treatment. Each responded beautifully. I took the bait and the hook was set. I used the techniques more and more with great success.

When the invitation was extended for me to join a research department at Michigan State University's College of Osteopathic Medicine, I jumped at the chance. Here was my opportunity to begin to demystify cranial osteopathy and perhaps understand the mechanisms of this system, which we were later to name the craniosacral system.

Hands-On Energy: Acupuncture Once Again

We had just arrived at our new home in East Lansing, Michigan, in a caravan consisting of two passenger cars and one large rental truck. While we were unloading the furniture, our realtor, Tomie, came by. She was a very nice lady who had been very accommodating in helping us to purchase the house. So when she asked if I would treat her right shoulder as soon as my treatment table was unloaded, I said yes, even though I wasn't really in the mood after having just spent two days driving a truck and another couple of hours moving furniture. She waited around for me to unload the table, though, so what could I do? She had me.

We went into the room that was to be a study of sorts. We set up the portable treatment table and she sat on it. I stood behind her, cupping my hands over her shoulders much as I had done for Harriet. Within seconds I could feel a line of heat develop in Tomie's right shoulder. It got hotter and hotter. It was precisely where the triple-heater meridian courses over the shoulder. This fact did not dawn on me at the time, though; I was very tired and sort of coasting.

I stood behind Tomie for perhaps fifteen minutes as the line of heat that traversed her right shoulder became uncomfortably hot. The heat built to a crescendo. I felt a lot of pain and burning across the palm of my hand, approximate to the line of heat. This discomfort lasted a minute or so. Tomie did some heavy breathing and perspiring. Suddenly everything got quiet. She smiled and said the pain was gone. My hand felt better. The treatment was obviously over. I didn't have the slightest idea what I had done to facilitate the therapeutic response, but I knew that I would try it again as soon as I had the chance.

I carried a red line, about a half-inch wide, across my palm for three days after this treatment. It felt like a sunburn, yet it didn't really bother me unless something came in contact with it; then it gave me a burning sensation. What had happened? In retrospect, I think I had experienced my first opening of an acupuncture meridian by hand. The timing was good for me because my fatigue had taken my left brain pretty much out of the way.

Tomie's shoulder never gave her another problem after that one treatment. That was June 1975. I saw her regularly, both as a patient and socially, until we left Michigan in December 1982. Tomie even visited with us in Florida over the Christmas holidays on three occasions after that. There was never any talk of right shoulder pain recurrence.

Pulling Energy Through the Meridians

Tomie's daughter, Sandy, was the next person to give me a lesson in the hands-on opening of acupuncture meridians. Sandy was an airline stewardess living in Ft. Lauderdale, Florida. She had awakened one Sunday morning in the fall of 1975 minus the use of her left arm. The arm and shoulder were painful and dysfunctional. She had seen a neurologist and was doing physiotherapy at his recommendation. He had not come up with any firm diagnosis, though, and she was not getting any better. She agreed to fly to Michigan if I would see her.

I treated Sandy each day for two weeks. I was into Kirlian photography at the time. The pictures of her fingers showed a much smaller energy output from the left hand than from the right. I did some acupuncture to reduce the pain. This was reasonably successful, but additional Kirlian photography showed that it did not equalize the energy output between her two hands, nor did it restore the strength to the left arm and hand. Sandy did not have enough strength to hold a full cup of water with her left hand. The oppositional strength of her thumb and fingers, as well as the wrist strength, were very much reduced.

After a couple of symptom-reducing acupuncture treatments, I did some structural corrections to the neck, upper back and ribs. (I didn't know anything about arcing as yet.)

I found myself wondering if hands-on energy work would be of any help. I held her left hand with my left hand in a handshake grip.

Her hand felt cold and relatively lifeless. I put my right hand around her wrist and just thought about the hand and wrist warming, vitalizing, and getting strong. Sure enough, some warming occurred. Then I got a sense that fluid or something was beginning to flow in the hand and wrist. I didn't say anything, nor did Sandy. We just sat for about five minutes, both of us feeling the changes.

Suddenly it dawned on me that I could feel the acupuncture meridians as they passed through her wrist. I concentrated on each meridian individually. It seemed that the greatest change and flow of fluid was on the palmar side of the wrist where the pericardial meridian conducts energy (chi). The origin of this meridian is in the pericardium of the chest, and it terminates at the end of the third finger. I thought it was a good meridian to provide revitalization to the arm and hand.

I began to mentally urge the meridian to flow. I also visualized an open connection between it and the triple-heater meridian, which returns chi energy centralward to the body. This seemed to work. Either consciously or nonconsciously, Sandy began to experiment with her hand. She began to move her fingers and tighten and loosen her grip. The warmth in her hand was improving quite remarkably.

I let my hands think for themselves. (This was before I knew they had more intelligence than my head.) Both of my hands went to Sandy's upper arm, where they fashioned a ring around it. I had my thumb tips touching on one side of the arm and my middle fingertips touching on the other side. I gradually began to "pull" energy from her shoulder into her arm as though my hands were magnetic. As this energy reached the point on her arm where my hands were placed, I slowly moved my hands further down toward her hand, carrying the sense of vitalization and energy with me. If I moved too fast, I lost contact with whatever it was I was pulling with me.

I reasoned that the pericardial, heart and lung meridians all conduct energy and vitalization away from the body, so I worked to open these meridians. The large intestine, triple heater, and small intestinal meridians all conduct from the hand to the trunk; therefore, I worked against them. I thought this approach would be okay because

I would essentially "back flush" these latter three meridians.

In any case, I kept my hands intact in the form of a ring and moved very slowly and painstakingly outward along the upper arm, careful to bring the sense of vitalization with me. I passed the elbow without difficulty and slowly began to move my hands down the forearm to the wrist.

At the wrist my hands decided to change their position. I felt like a privileged spectator to what my hands were doing. My right hand arranged itself longitudinally so that it covered the back of Sandy's wrist and hand. My left hand did the same thing on the inside of her wrist. It essentially looked like a sandwich, with Sandy's hand the filling and my two hands the slices of bread. The middle fingers of my two hands were parallel to the triple heater and pericardial meridians.

In my mind's eye, I began to pull away from Sandy's body with my left hand, which was on the inner surface of her hand, while I pushed towards her with my right hand, positioned on the back of her hand. There was some perceived resistance for awhile. Then suddenly there was an opening and a softening and a flowing, and every other good thing you can think of. Immediately after what I would now call a "release," Sandy smiled. I took my hands away and she felt "normal."

I redid the Kirlian photographs. Her hands were close to equal. I shot a picture of my own fingers, as well, and there was corona energy going all over the place.

All this took place on Friday, at the end of the first week. I continued to see Sandy daily during the second week, but this was more for me than it was for her arm and hand. She was fine and remained fine. I have no idea what caused this to happen to Sandy. Perhaps it occurred because I needed to learn another lesson. Thank you, Sandy.

Our Bodies Are Our Own Best Laboratories

The V-Spread

It was the fall of 1978. Our research had been going quite success-
fully at Michigan State University. The concepts of the PressureStat
Model, energy cysts, direction of energy, and SomatoEmotional
Release were all falling pretty well into place.

I was at home one day pruning some rather large shrubs. As I
trimmed one branch, the cut end rebounded directly into the cornea
of my left eye. It took all I could do to keep from yelling hysterically
and running around the yard like a maniac. I reasoned with myself and
felt a little more stable and objective about the situation. I opened
my injured left eye. Everything was a total blur. I could see light, but
I was sure that I had damaged the cornea. I'd never before had a sensation like this.

Finally I went into the house and asked my wife to look at my eye.
She said there was a big dent in the shape of a 'Y' laying on its side that
went across my pupil. I realized how much I did not want my cornea
to be damaged and my vision impaired. I thought about seeing an
ophthalmologist or going to the emergency room, but it all seemed
like too much to think about. I knew what they would do, and I did not
want it.

I suddenly heard myself say, "Hey, dipsh__, you teach the V-spread
all the time. If you really believe in it, why not try it on yourself?" I
went into the bedroom and laid down on the bed. I looked at my
watch; it was 1:50 P.M. I made a 'V' with my left index and middle fingers and positioned the eyeball in the "crotch" of the 'V.' I experimented
around the back of my head with my right hand to find a position
that felt right for sending the energy. Once I found it, I used my index,
middle and ring fingers to send energy from this locus through my
left eyeball. After a minute or two I could feel energy building. My
eyeball began pulsating and it hurt a lot for what seemed like forever.
I thought it probably wouldn't work. The eye pain got worse, but I

kept on with the V-spread "just because." All of a sudden there was a pop in my eyeball—which I was sure could be heard in the other room. Immediately after the pop occurred, the pain left. The blurred vision cleared. My anxiety disappeared. I was filled with elation. It had worked! My eye was okay.

I went into the living room and found my wife. She had not heard the pop, but she said that the dent in my cornea was gone.

My confidence in energy direction as a therapeutic modality—and as a real phenomenon—was bolstered several hundred percent. I thanked the bush for cooperating. I also thanked whomever it is that composes these scenarios when they seem appropriate. I was a different person after this experience. I could really teach the direction of energy with no holds barred. What a beautiful experience!

My Experiences With CO_2-O_2 Inhalation

During a two-day seminar in February 1980 at the Continuing Medical Education Center in Pontiac, Michigan, Dr. June MacRae and I arranged to do some preliminary investigation into the effects of CO_2 inhalation upon the function of the craniosacral system. The investigation centered around the work of Dr. Meduna at the University of Illinois. He had developed a therapy wherein patients inhaled a mixture of twenty to thirty percent carbon dioxide combined with oxygen. It was used for neuroses and various dysfunctions such as stuttering and nervous tics.

The question of a possible relationship between Dr. Meduna's approach and CranioSacral Therapy occurred to me while I was reading his case histories. The clinical courses of many of my CranioSacral Therapy patients seemed to parallel those of many of his CO_2-O_2-treated patients. The obvious question was: Does CO_2-O_2 inhalation affect the craniosacral system and its function?

In order to explore this question, it initially seemed reasonable to rely upon my subjective impression of craniosacral system events—as transmitted through my hands from the subjects during the course of several CO_2-O_2 mixture inhalations. After manually monitoring the craniosacral system function of five different subjects, I was satisfied that the inhalation of CO_2-O_2 mixture did result in spontaneous release of craniosacral system restrictions. There was also a marked increase in craniosacral amplitude with less membranous resistance to motion.

The gas mixture in these initial trials was thirty percent CO_2 with seventy percent O_2. It was administered by a mask and breathing bag in a closed ventilatory system. Most subjects took three to five inhalations of the gas mixture followed by a rest of about three to four minutes. We repeated this cycle about ten times for each subject. (One subject took fifteen deep breaths on one occasion. He had previous experience with CO_2-O_2 inhalation.)

My impression while monitoring these subjects was that progressive craniosacral system corrections were accomplished as the sets of inhalations were repeated for each person. The craniosacral system seemed progressively more relaxed and easy in its motion after each set of inhalations. After two or three rest periods, the craniosacral system began to produce its own still points. These occurrences were followed by marked and significant releases of membranous restriction with spontaneous correction of a variety of motion distortions. I am convinced that to achieve similar corrections using the manual approach might have taken several minutes, if not hours, of treatment time.

Since I was considering the use of CO_2-O_2 inhalation with Cranio-Sacral Therapy for brain-dysfunctioning children, the sixth subject had to be me. I would not apply the CO_2-O_2 treatment in these cases without first experiencing it.

My first inhalation of CO_2-O_2 gas mixture seemed generally acceptable to my body, but exhalation was somewhat difficult. The second inhalation was rather tenuous but was achievable. The second exhalation was not possible at first; my chest would not allow it. I finally exhaled a little bit. As a result of my failure to exhale completely, the volume of my third inhalation was significantly reduced. After the third inhalation the mask was removed. I had great difficulty fully exhaling—but what a relief to have that mask off my face!

During this first CO_2-O_2 breathing experience, I had a visual hallucination of an orange background with white polka dots. I vividly recalled a near-drowning incident that occurred when I was about ten years old. I was at Olsen's Beach in St. Clair Shores, Michigan. I was there with my friend Gordon, who was a better swimmer than I. We decided to swim out to the end of the dock where the water was about six or eight feet deep. I couldn't make it and was floundering, but no one paid any attention because they all thought I could swim. The water was very brown and murky. My reflexes were trying to make me exhale, but I was underwater and knew if I exhaled I would have to inhale, and then I would drown. I vividly recalled my respiratory system bucking, trying to stop me from exhaling—just as was happening during the CO_2-O_2 inhalations.

Gordon finally saw my plight and yelled for help. Some larger boys pulled me out of the water, laid me on my stomach on the dock, and proceeded to further prevent me from breathing by awkwardly applying artificial respiration. I recalled them pushing the air out of my lungs while I was trying to take air in—exactly the same feeling I had during the CO_2-O_2 inhalations.

Another memory I had was of the ether anesthesia I received for my tonsillectomy at age four. I remembered the doctor saying he was pouring water on the mask. That "water" smelled terrible. I fought as hard as I could. I couldn't really breathe. I wondered why they wanted to kill me. Where was my mother and, even more significantly, where was my father? I was so scared.

That night following the CO_2-O_2 inhalations, I had very clear dreams of the near-drowning incident. Then I dreamed that I removed my sternal plate, as one would during an autopsy, and threw it away. I felt much lighter but more vulnerable. I had mixed feelings. I did not want to completely discard my sternum. It was my defense, my armor. I took it out and put it back several times. I don't know where my sternum was when I awakened at 5:30 A.M.

A few days later, back in my office in East Lansing, I had a strong desire to inhale more CO_2-O_2. It was as though something needed to go to completion. I called Dr. MacRae and she agreed to work further with me. This time my breathing was better, but I still bucked a lot and had difficulty with exhalation. I then recalled being hit in the solar plexus and not being able to breathe. My rib cage just wouldn't move.

It was my first year playing high school football. I was lying on the ground. The coach looked at me rather disdainfully and commented that I was okay. "Just had the wind knocked out of you." I was mortified. I couldn't move for what seemed like hours. I'm sure the memory was a CO_2-O_2-induced SomatoEmotional Release.

After re-experiencing this memory I did better with the CO_2-O_2 but still had some difficulty with full exhalation. Dr. MacRae suggested that we add one inhalation to a set to obtain better relaxation. It helped, and I could inhale deeper and exhale more fully because I knew that my next breath would be without the mask. I felt safer and more in control.

After a deep inhalation I felt like I had a rod in my spine. My body felt fairly relaxed around this rod. Dr. MacRae suggested that this sensation was symbolic of my accepting too much responsibility for others. After some conversation she helped me to realize that the only one who could make me accept the responsibility for others was me. She suggested that God was ultimately responsible for everyone. I was not God, therefore I did not need to allow others to be dependent upon me. I then realized that I asked for this dependency. When I got what I asked for, I rebelled against it because it got too heavy. This is probably a syndrome shared by many physicians.

I envisioned a lead bar placed diagonally across my sternum after the second to last inhalation of CO_2-O_2 that day. That night I dreamed a lot and realized that several events had created a weight on my chest.

At the time of my father's death, I had just turned fourteen. I was awakened from a sound sleep by my mother calling me. My father, whom I loved dearly, was lying on the couch and my mother was rubbing his chest. She told me to telephone Dr. Cross. I could not discern the letters in the phone directory; I had lost my ability to read. In a panic, Mother screamed at me and left my father to come and call the doctor herself. My father was dead when the fire department arrived. I was totally confused. I accepted responsibility for my father's death. I loved him so much. It was my fault that he died that night.

At my father's funeral I was sobbing uncontrollably and could not get my breath. (It felt just like my experience with the CO_2-O_2 inhalations.) Someone told me after the funeral that I was now the man of the family. I was responsible for taking care of my mother. I couldn't remember the face of the person but I could hear his voice. I felt very afraid and inadequate.

I questioned the minister at our church as to why my father was taken by this "loving God." The minister lost patience with my questions and told me to go away and not return to the church until I was able to restore my faith in God and accept his works. I never went back.

All of these factors became clear in my dreams that night—after this further work with the CO_2-O_2 inhalations. By morning it was clear to me that I did, in fact, accept responsibility and solicit the dependency of others. When it got too heavy, I rebelled. This may have caused some of the dependent people to become angry and hurt by my refusal to continue to accept their dependence. The thought of this made me feel guilty. Perhaps I played god because I thought I would be better at it than God, who I believed had so cruelly taken my father. All of this had made my rib cage immobile so that I couldn't breathe properly.

It was over. When I walked to work that morning, my ribs were snapping and cracking with pleasure as they mobilized. I was breathing deeply like a child. I had found a new toy—breath. I began to run without getting short of breath. I had been short-winded since I was a teenager. I had given up basketball and did not go out for track because of this short-windedness. Instead I played football, hockey and lifted weights.

It is wondrous the way events shape our lives. Had I not developed the neurotic pattern now clear to me, I probably would not be an osteopathic physician today. I probably would not be considering the effect of CO_2-O_2 inhalation upon the craniosacral system. Thank you, again, whoever you are.

Reincarnation? What Next?

In July 1978 French osteopath Jean-Pierre Barral told me that I had some spasm of the left ureter. In July 1979 he told me the same thing. The closest condition I had to this that I knew of was a recurring case of shingles that appeared when I was under a lot of stress. I controlled it by self-acupuncture.

In January 1980, while visiting us in Michigan, Jean-Pierre examined me using his "off the body" method, which uses heat or energy patterns to determine the age of a person's injury or illness. He told me that there was an abnormal heat pattern over the left part of my abdomen. After moving his hands about for a few minutes, his face took on an expression of disbelief and his voice a tone of marked astonishment. Finally he said, "John, this is an injury from one hundred and forty years ago!" (That would be the year 1840.)

As he spoke I remembered an experience prior to our move to Michigan in 1975. A friend and I were playing around with hypnoregression. As the subject, I saw myself as a black male slave in Charleston, South Carolina. I had decided to run away. The first night after my escape I hid in a farmer's barn. The next morning I awakened to find him standing over me, about to plunge a pitchfork into my body. I died of fright before he stabbed me in the upper left abdomen. As I died, I flew up above and watched the anger of the farmer as he plunged the pitchfork into my vacated body. I laughed at him derisively.

I recalled this incident as Jean-Pierre worked with me non-verbally. I again saw the angry farmer, so controlled and driven by his emotions, prejudices and hatred, acting so inhumanely against another human being. Suddenly, though, I felt total compassion for the farmer. I realized that my attitude of derision was deplorable. I hope that one day I can see this farmer once more and perhaps help him to shed his negative emotions. Who knows, maybe we have already met again since 1840! Thank you, Jean-Pierre.

Can it be that we carry trauma from one life to another? Since this experience I have come to believe that we do. I also feel sure that we carry these traumas with us when the circumstances of death reflect an unacceptable resolution. My attitude of derision as the farmer stabbed me with the pitchfork was an unacceptable end to that life. I understand that now, and the symptoms are no longer with me. Since Jean-Pierre's evaluation and my resolution of this "experience," I have had no further recurrence of my shingles, and Jean-Pierre no longer sees my ureter as a problem—at least he hasn't mentioned it lately.

Other Insights, Other Questions

During the latter part of April 1980, I felt a powerful restlessness and dissatisfaction building up inside of me.

In early May I went to Crystal River, Florida, to participate in the presentation of a seminar for the Florida Academy of Osteopathy. The other two lecturers were osteopaths Dick MacDonald and Herb Miller. I recall telling Dick that life felt like doing thirty days in jail: It was boring, I knew it would be over soon, and I wished it would hurry up. Dick became a little angry with my dissatisfaction. He believed I had a lot of work yet to do, while I thought I had done it all.

After the seminar was over, Dick offered to give me a treatment. Within a very short time of sitting down on the table, I went into a position in which the top of my head was on the floor and my buttocks were still on the table. I was slightly hyperextended, to say the least, but it felt right. I was feeling releases that I never dreamed could happen. Pains and dysfunctions that I had carried with me for a lot of years were popping loose.

Then we went into the recall of a very specific injury I incurred when I was an eleventh-grader. It was the first football game of the season, and I was the starting linebacker. On our first defensive play a hole opened on my side of the line and a huge fullback barreled through. I put my head down and charged him like a bull. I remember a big noise when my helmet hit his thigh pad. I came back to consciousness in the fourth quarter of the game, over an hour later. I was able to walk and talk, but I didn't know what day it was or how many fingers the coach was holding up. I had total amnesia from the time of the tackle until I asked my friend Richard where I was.

I had often wondered why I'd been out of it for so long. During the treatment with Dick, I completely relived the experience. I hit the ball carrier's right thigh pad with the front of my helmet. My head snapped back and I almost broke my neck. I could feel my head rotate slightly to the left. In a play-by-play sequence, I felt my head hyperextend on my atlas, the cervical vertebrae hyperextend one by one from upper to lower, the upper thoracics hyperextend one by one down to the fifth, and so forth. I also felt a very sharp, sickening pain in the left knee. I had not remembered any of this before.

After the treatment I had a lot of aches and pains for a few days, but it all felt right. During my recall of the collision with the ball carrier, I felt a lot of energy go into my head. By the end of the treatment this energy was radiating out of my right forehead. This radiation continued for the rest of that day and about halfway through the next. I began to feel softer, less critical. My wife and children were astonished at the personality change I exhibited when I returned home from the seminar. I was tolerant of mistakes and errors. I was less arrogant and far more reasonable.

Accepting Trauma for Another

The year was 1936. I was about four years old and was playing in front of our home on Cadillac Avenue in Detroit, Michigan. The four-lane street was rather busy, even in those days. There was a little girl, probably six or seven years old, who lived across the street. We used to shout to each other across the street in an attempt to be friends. Neither of us was allowed to cross to the other side.

It so happened that one summer morning, as we were shouting across to each other, we began to move closer and closer to the street in order hear better. Because neither her nor my parents were in view, it was finally decided that one of us should cross the street so we could play together. Since she was the older of the two of us, she got the task. She ran across the street between the cars.

She wasn't in my yard very long, though, before she became frightened that her mother would discover she had broken the rules by coming over to see me. I remember vividly that she sort of panicked and ran into the street. As she reached the other side she was hit just above the right knee by a car. She flew up in the air, landed on the car's fender, then fell off into the street. The noise of a horn and screeching brakes brought mothers out of houses all up and down the street. The girl had fallen on the far side of the car, so I couldn't see her. A man picked her up and carried her into another car and they drove away. I never saw her again.

The police came and there was a lot of confusion. I felt terribly guilty that she had come over to see me and had been hit by a car. The police asked me, of all people, how fast the car was going when it hit the girl. I said, "Thirty-five miles per hour," because I'd heard my father mention that speed once while he was driving us somewhere. I really had no idea how fast the car was going. I hoped that I hadn't gotten the man who was driving the car in trouble; he was crying.

One day in 1983 Dick MacDonald and I were trading treatments. He had me begin my session in a standing position. I felt pain in my right knee. Then my knee buckled. I went sideways onto the table, then fell over the other side. Nothing like this had ever happened to me, but it felt very real and the releases were very powerful. Suddenly I completely recalled the incident I described above. I let go of a lot of energy, pain, fear and guilt. I let go of some more responsibility that day, too.

From this experience, it appears that it is possible to absorb an injury inflicted upon another person to whom you may be connected—emotionally, spiritually, by circumstance, or whatever. Perhaps I took on the girl's injury because I felt it was my fault that she was hit by a car. Since I never saw her again, I suspect that she was killed.

Learning From Advanced Classes at the Institute

The Advanced Class in CranioSacral Therapy has become, over the years, an extremely important learning laboratory for me, as well as for ninety-nine percent of my trainees. There are many reasons for this, not the least of which is the practice session that takes place in the last hour or two of the final day. It has become my habit at that time to give my body to the ten-person group for evaluation and treatment.

I Discover My Own Birth

In January 1988, as I lay on the table, I experienced a sense of complete trust as Susan, the elected chief therapist, directed the placement of the other nine pairs of hands upon my body. I made little or no conscious attempt to analyze the process. It was very natural and easy to give myself over to it. Within just a few minutes I began to vaguely move in and out of a sensation of birth. The sensation slowly solidified, and I could feel the hands of William Naggs, M.D., on my head assisting the delivery process. My neck retracted. The therapist holding my head commented on the phenomenon. For just an instant I felt like a turtle pulling back into my shell. I then seemed to use my shoulders and arms against the inner rim of the birth canal to resist the doctor's pulling. Dr. Naggs was trying to help, but I didn't see it that way.

Susan asked me something about why I didn't want to be born. That was not the issue. I became aware that the doctor was working against the natural delivery process, with good but misguided intention. I wanted to go slower so that the process would be in keeping with nature's plan.

I shared this with Susan (I believe it was her) and she very wisely suggested that I tell the doctor to stop pulling and let nature take its course. I did and he honored my request. (After all, this was my fantasy.) For an indefinite but considerable amount of time, I experienced the most remarkable and pleasant twisting and untwisting, relaxing, and lengthening of my neck, torso and, finally, my legs. It felt like my first, and to date most pleasant, spinal manipulation treatment. (No offense to those wonderful people who have applied their therapeutic skills to my body.) I now fully support Dick MacDonald's statement that the natural delivery process is a person's first spinal treatment. It is also the initiation to CranioSacral Therapy.

The process went slowly, unhurried by the doctor's pullings and urgings. I'm sure that the reality of my birth experience was being changed here at my request. My body lengthened and unwound beautifully. It gave me a beautiful experience as I left the safety of the womb to enter the outside world. A most remarkable sensation came over me as one of the therapists (Scott) placed a fist on my back. He seemed to be pushing down quite hard. This felt like my mother's pubic region. Once I got past this point there were no further problems to overcome.

One of the assistant therapists (Scott, I believe) then asked if I'd had any problems with my heart or breathing at my delivery. I knew of none and did not feel that there had been any at the time. Next I felt what seemed to be about four hands and a forearm begin to firmly press on the front of my rib cage. As this was happening I saw an image of my father. He was at the delivery of his son, yet he was sad and tearful. I suddenly realized that my birth reminded him of the wife he'd had before my mother. She had borne him two daughters and then died of cancer. He then married my mother and they conceived me. (I was born on February 10, 1932.)

I saw that my father still loved his deceased wife very much. I felt so much compassion for him that I accepted his grief into my body in order to help him. (The lungs are the organs of grief in Chinese medicine, as you may recall.) As I imagined this, his countenance visibly brightened and his posture straightened. I realized that I would take his grief and deal with it later in my own life—a lot of reasoning for a newborn, but it was very clear to me.

Then a most remarkable realization occurred as the therapists helped me to release the lung-based grief from my chest. I knew that I was meant to be born to my father and his first wife. Her death by cancer was not anticipated. She was twenty-eight years old when she died. Since it was determined that he would be my father, another mother had to be found for me. My mother had never quite fit into the arrangement for as long as I could remember. Now I knew why: She was a second choice. Father loved her very much, but it just wasn't quite the same. What an insight this was for me.

I slowly returned to awareness of the here and now. I was amazed to realize that an hour and forty-five minutes had passed. It was a beautiful experience. I felt wonderful and still do. It's really difficult to question the therapeutic process when experiences like this are released from your memory banks. What a wonderful lesson.

News From Outer Space

The next Advanced-class treatment opened more doors for me. After the trainees placed their hands on me, the chief therapist (Stan) began to gently but persistently push me into imagery and dialogue. I quite consistently saw a black background with purple areas. I had thoughts about accepting my father's grief and about many past experiences with SomatoEmotional Release. My left brain would not be quiet. Stan persisted.

I saw myself on our front porch swing at 5706 Cadillac Avenue one night studying Dad's red neon "Notary Public" sign. He was teaching me how to look at it from the inside out. Mom wanted me in bed. If I kept staring at the sign, however, I wouldn't have to go to bed. I saw a black border with a purple center. Soon a shiny spot developed in the purple center. It was like a purple-violet radiant crystal. With some urging from Stan, the crystal came closer and became larger. It turned silver. I kept looking at the silver area. Then I saw a face in it that looked like a porpoise.

Without hesitation Stan asked me the "porpoise" (purpose) of that face. I was amused and relaxed by his play on words. The humor he injected seemed to ease the barrier I was struggling against. The porpoise face turned into a spaceship, which had a voice. It began to communicate, first with me and then with the rest of the group through me. The points of discussion, which I remember so well, were:

1. The occupants weren't quite sure whether I was ready to receive what they were going to communicate to me.

2. I was one of them but had been assigned to earth for about five thousand years, during which time I had experienced many lives. They told me that I should not get caught up in the earthly life, however. Instead, I must always recognize that I am an envoy from beyond.

3. My assignment from the beginning of my time on earth was to "soften" the earth's inhabitants. One of the ways this is being accomplished now is through teaching "soft touch" in workshops such as CranioSacral Therapy and ShareCare® (a one-day workshop for laypeople). Workshops such as these help to allay fear and reduce anger and frustration. Soft touch promotes love and union.

4. We come from infinity, far beyond any present-day conceptual scientific framework we've established here on earth.

5. The God of earthlings is a subsidiary of the God of the Universe. Earthlings' concepts of the universe are diminutive compared to what is really out there.

6. Our planet is like a person. It is our mother. The softening of earth people through soft touch and love will cause Mother Earth to be loved and respected by those she supports. She deserves love and respect. She gives so unselfishly and without question, but her gifts are running out.

I knew this time around that my mother had given me toughness and my father compassion—both necessary for this task.

I was asked by the chief therapist if there were others present from the same place. With my eyes closed, I pointed around one of the therapists to a table on the other side of the room where they told me Stan's wife had just come in and laid down.

I don't know what this experience means, but it was sobering and wondrous.

A Past Life

In a session three months later, I began to see images almost as soon as the ten pairs of hands were upon me in a gentle, energy-providing way. First I saw and felt as though I was in a cylinder made of Lucite or some other transparent material. I was very calm and felt that everything was going as it was supposed to. Then I was ejected from the cylinder as if propelled from a torpedo tube. I headed through space toward planet Earth. I circled a few times and came down some distance from a castle fortress, complete with a moat and drawbridge. The building was teeming with barbarians. I was off a distance in some trees and they had not seen me.

I looked down at myself and realized I was in the wrong uniform. I wanted to go into the fortress, blend in and be inconspicuous. I had on a rather snappy-looking, Nazi officer-type uniform. I found I had the ability to change my clothing by thought, so I changed my uniform to more closely match the raggedy-looking ones the soldiers were wearing. I needed to get closer to make myself and my garb more appropriate, but I couldn't see the details from this distance. I began to walk toward the barbarians until I got very close. At this point my concern over the proper attire and demeanor faded away because I realized that the soldiers still couldn't see me. I was invisible. I entered the castle fortress and looked around at the soldiers milling about. Many were chewing meat off bones. They were talking loudly and sometimes waving the bones at each other. "Hussars" was the name that came to mind when the therapists asked who these people were.

We were somewhere in Eastern Europe. It was late afternoon. It was rather cold. Snow patches were here and there. Upon looking around, I realized this was not going to be a good place for me to do my work, so I left. I was invisible so I just flew away. It was beautiful. I notified my home base that I was changing locations. I seemed to soar effortlessly around the earth a few times, then I saw a sign that read "Tennessee" on a white background in the shape of that state. It was on a continent that looked like North America.

I went to Tennessee. As I approached, the maplike image turned realistic. I landed on a battlefield, where I became a Tennessee volunteer soldier. I had a bandage wrapped around my left shoulder and upper body. There was a lot of blood. I knew that I had a musket ball lodged against my upper ribs and shoulder joint. I elected to stay in this situation. A Yankee Civil War surgeon was preparing to remove the musket ball from my body. He had a cautery iron in the fire, which would be used to sterilize the wound after he took the musket ball out of my armpit. I felt detached. I knew that if I wanted to gather information about the strange fascination earth inhabitants seem to have with pain, I would have to experience this pain and see what was so enjoyable about it.

As I was imagining the musket ball being removed, the therapists were delivering a large energy cyst from my left armpit. The synchronization of the two events was perfect. Then the imaged surgeon sterilized my wound with the red-hot cautery iron. I got no joy from any of this. I remained puzzled about why earth people continue to do things like this to each other.

I reported my experience and impressions to my home base and returned to an outpost for repairs and rejuvenation. The mission was a failure. I was trying to discover why earth people continue to inflict and suffer pain, destruction and death. Reason told me that there must be some joy involved in it. But as I experienced the pain of the musket ball being removed and the cautery iron being applied, my earthly body felt no joy or satisfaction. I still don't understand.

Ramus Gives a Tune-Up

I received my next Advanced-class treatment in September 1988. It was a very quiet, rejuvenating experience. During the five-day class, one of the students (Toni) presented a guide named Ramus for her treatments. He became so prominent during the class that the group elected him chief therapist. He was therefore in charge of my treatment.

Ramus instructed the class to put healing, no-strings-attached, generic energy into my body. As this went on, I felt that Ramus was scanning my skeletal structure for chips, dents and weak spots and then repairing them. He seemed to do the same with my muscles, ligaments and tendons. He did not do anything with my viscera. (It was not verbalized, but I sensed that visceral healing was not appropriate at that time.) It was a wonderful, quiet, non-sensational experience. I felt serene when it was over, as if I had been oiled, greased, overhauled, and tuned up.

A Gorilla Speaks

The next Advanced class, in November 1988, gave me a very nice recharging treatment. My chief therapist (Chris) asked my Inner Physician to please come forward. A huge, wonderful, kind, gentle, and absolutely non-threatening gorilla appeared.

He said I should not forget that I was one of his descendants. He reminded me that I had wondered for some time what purpose grazing animals, such as wildebeest, reindeer and caribou, serve on this planet. They eat grass and fertilize to grow more grass, but what does all this contribute to the ecosystem? He explained that all grazing herds are producers of positive thought forms. Their product is necessary to counterbalance the negative thought forms produced by so many humans and some other predatory animals. That was our lesson for the day.

Reynaldo and Umberto

The Advanced class in May 1989 treated me very well. Shari was the chief therapist. I had two guides present themselves during my session. Reynaldo and Umberto were their names.

Reynaldo was very serious. He let me know that I had much work to do. I was to study the motivation behind violence and the destructive activities in which so many earth people indulge. He told me that the work done so far was good, but if the earth was to be salvaged there was not much time to waste.

Umberto, on the other hand, was insistent that we all have some fun. We needed to dance and drink wine. He said that he, Shari and I had lived together in Florence. We were all lovers and partners. We shared a wonderful life at that time.

This seemed to be a lesson in balance between serious work and real fun.

Confirmation and Expansion

My experience in the July 1989 Advanced class was of confirmation and expansion. While I was on the table I began to make pronouncements to the class that came out of who knows where.

My chief therapist (Lisa) went a little fast in the beginning. I offered no resistance. She said she had never treated a "no-resistance" patient before. She didn't know quite what to do, so she talked. Once we were past that, I began to speak.

In essence, I said the following:

1. There are specific nuclei in the human brain that are activated by violent, destructive and homicidal behaviors. It is a similar phenomenon to thrill-seeking. When activated, these nuclei give a sense of pleasure and gratification.

2. CranioSacral Therapy stimulates the development of brain nuclei that balance the effect of these violence-responding nuclei. There is more to CranioSacral Therapy than touch and structure. The energy input positively affects chromosomal development and control. It stimulates the development of these "loving behavior" nuclei.

3. The pleasure produced by violent, destructive and homicidal behaviors is tempered and modulated by CranioSacral Therapy. Further, balancing nuclei develop that produce pleasure from doing loving activities.

4. It all fits together with an evolving chromosomal modification that is in process.

5. If the negative energy level becomes high enough, the surface of the earth could and would spontaneously incinerate. Although we are not near that level at present, we must not become complacent.

The process is working and the level of joy derived from violent and destructive behaviors is topping off. We must continue the work.

Closing

In this chapter I have shared with you some very personal experiences that have made an impact on my life and development. I'm not trying to convince you of anything, just reporting my experiences. You can make of them what you wish. I do hope this sharing helps to open your mind as these experiences have opened mine. Once the mind is open, it seems that things begin to happen that cause further opening. It is as though the powers that be see a chink in our armor and know we are thereafter more and more amenable to further opening.

I do not possess the meaning of my experiences. I am comfortable with the realization that there is a tremendous amount of stuff out there that I don't know about. I hope to increase your comfort level with this same realization.

Chapter Six

Channeling

For therapeutic facilitators who work with characterizations such as Inner Physicians, Higher Consciousness and Inner Wisdom, there is an excellent chance they will encounter a situation that sounds and feels like they are in communication with an entity outside the client's immediate and personal consciousness. Some call it "channeling." That is, they may feel as if they are speaking with a discarnate guide who is involved with the client on an esoteric or spiritual level. If you are one who needs facts in order to believe an occurrence of this nature, you will have difficulty with this because to verify such a situation is well nigh impossible.

Arguments can be made that the "spirit guide" is a figment of the client's imagination. Similarly, any clinical changes that might occur after conversations and encounters between therapeutic facilitators and spirit guides might well be the result of suggestion, therapeutic imagery, or the like. On the other hand, phenomena sometimes occur that make it so difficult for facilitators to explain in non-spiritual terms what they have witnessed that it seems more rational to entertain a spiritual guide explanation rather than continue to stretch logic in order to maintain a more traditional or scientific frame of mind.

In the final analysis, it is up to each client and therapeutic facilitator team to determine whether or not they believe there has been contact and assistance from a spiritual entity. I believe it matters little what the personal belief system of the therapeutic facilitator allows.

I suggest to practitioners that they make it a rule not to disagree with any belief system or circumstance a client presents, so long as it rings true and is verified with the craniosacral rhythm (when it is used as a significance detector). I try to blend with patients, becoming part of them, leaving my personal beliefs and prejudices outside the treatment room door.

I know I can't cop out that easily on questions about channeling, but suspension of my belief system is my personal code of therapeutic facilitator conduct. As for my beliefs, I think it is best to describe some experiences that have influenced my present feelings about such matters. You may then better understand the how and why of my belief system. I described some of my personal experiences in Chapter Five. Those that I am about to recount all occurred while I was in the role of therapeutic facilitator.

Frederick, Doctor of Internal Medicine, Calls in a Consultant

It was during a session marked by deep relaxation coupled with intense concentration that my first experience with a patient's discarnate spiritual guide occurred. The year was 1984. The patient was a very pleasant, middle-aged woman who was a practicing psychologist/psychotherapist. She had been in chronic pain in the left arm, shoulder, upper back, neck, and head since an automobile accident two years earlier. She had run the gamut of the therapeutic spectrum: orthopedics, physical therapy, chiropractic and biofeedback. I did not find a structural basis for her pain, but there seemed to be excessive retention of multiple, traumatically induced energy cysts.

As we were working with the energy cyst release process—combined with some SomatoEmotional Release of materials that predated the automobile accident—I enlisted the aid of her Inner Physician, who came forward in a very helpful and accommodating manner.

The Inner Physician was named Frederick. He confirmed for us when the precise body positions for energy cyst releases were achieved. He told us when the maximum release from a given position had been attained. And he informed us that a lot of the traumatic energy that remained from the automobile accident was due to retained resentment and smoldering anger over the dissolution six years earlier of the patient's twenty-two-year marriage.

As I worked with the patient and Frederick over a half-dozen sessions, my relationship with Frederick became more and more cordial and relaxed. (The patient was totally unaware of our conversations.) Frederick let me know that the end of the pain syndrome would not occur until the ill feelings about the marriage had been completely resolved. I continued to ask Frederick how we could best achieve this final release of resentment and anger. He gave some advice but seemed a little vague and unsure of himself as we continued our attempt to resolve feelings from the divorce. Our efforts in this direction were not totally successful.

During the sixth session I asked Frederick if there might be a consultant available whom he could invite into our conversations—one who might be willing and able to advise us regarding the last residuum of the pain syndrome and the related resentment and anger. As a rather experienced psychologist/psychotherapist, the patient was not easily moved toward total resolution of the ill will she continued to harbor against her ex-husband. She had her defenses well in place. She had tolerated several episodes of his unfaithfulness and philandering. The thanks she got for her tolerance (which is often enabling behavior in disguise) was that her husband finally asked for a divorce. This really hurt her pride and gave her a chance to develop an unhealthy level of self-righteous anger and lust for revenge.

When we asked for a consultant to come forward, the patient's voice became very deep and developed an accent I could not identify. It was a little difficult to understand. The new voice announced his name was EUPHEMUS. He spelled it for me. (Throughout this section, I use uppercase letters for the names of spirit guides to differentiate them from the names of Inner Physicians, Inner Wisdom and Tumors.) He was not of her nonconscious; rather, he had been "assigned" to help her deal with a problem that had been plaguing her for several hundred years. EUPHEMUS further explained that he had guided her to me because he knew I was "open" and would allow him and others to work through me.

I decided to go along with the scenario. I asked EUPHEMUS whether we had known each other before. He exclaimed, "Certainly! How could you have forgotten our time together, both in ancient Greece and Egypt?" I kept my wits about me and reminded the slightly insulted EUPHEMUS that I was earthbound at present. According to the way things work here on earth, I had amnesia of my previous spiritual existences and, in large part, of my previous earth incarnations. EUPHEMUS apologized for having forgotten how things worked on earth. He would keep this in mind and be patient with me.

EUPHEMUS said we had been healers together in Egypt. Before that, he had known of me in Greece, where I was a rather precocious and rebellious young healer in training. He told me that I was well-known throughout the Mediterranean world during the fourth century B.C. In fact, I was too well-known. I had demonstrated my talents without discretion. Thus, I was beheaded at the age of twelve by politically oriented and envious teachers. EUPHEMUS told me that three of the principal teachers who were responsible for my death were on earth right now, and they would like to repeat my decapitation. He told me I was not in any great danger at the present, but I should beware of jealousy and exercise caution. I thanked EUPHEMUS for the advice. I assured him I would be alert for danger and changed the subject back to the patient.

According to EUPHEMUS, this patient had been on Atlantis. During that incarnation she had been responsible in part for a certain man's loss of reputation, attendant shame, and ultimate demise. That man was her current ex-husband. EUPHEMUS explained that the patient needed to recognize that the disagreement and vengeful attitude between her and her ex-husband had been going on over many, many earth lifetimes. The problems would continue until both of them were willing to accept equal responsibility for their ongoing problems and to forget vengeance. It would go on until this patient accepted the fact that what her ex-husband had done was unimportant in the grand scheme of things. Then and only then would there be no further need for the pain that had brought her to see me.

I asked EUPHEMUS how I might promote resolution between these two souls. He instructed me to gradually enlighten this patient so that her tolerance for hearing the reasons for her symptoms would increase. He warned me not to tell her too much all at once. I broached the subject after she returned to conscious awareness. The patient was very receptive and seemed willing to work on the resolution of a problem that had begun several millennia before in Atlantis. I had three more sessions with the patient after this initial conversation with EUPHEMUS. She got complete relief of pain.

EUPHEMUS encouraged me to continue to be open. He also told me "they" would be using my services a lot more now that I was open. He bade me good-bye for awhile and told me not to worry. I was doing as they would like me to do. He also told me that he thought this patient could resolve the rest of her problem with their help. He did not anticipate that she would require any more of my services, but if another obstacle proved difficult, he would see to it that she returned to me. About six months later she returned for two mundane visits during which I mostly did energy work with her liver and the second and fourth chakra energy centers. There was no contact with EUPHEMUS. She is doing fine now.

I really did not know what to make of this experience, so I did not reject or accept it as being literally true. I could have made a case for psychology, painting this as a scenario of forgiveness with pride and dignity, but I felt as though I would be reaching in an attempt to stay on familiar ground. So I decided not to decide, but rather to remain open and see what might happen next.

THEO and the Actress

Four days after my final communication with EUPHEMUS, an actress in her mid-sixties came in. She complained of fainting and dizziness. She had suffered these symptoms for some fifteen years. Of late, the symptoms had worsened to the point that they interfered with her ability to perform. She feared she might stagger or faint while on stage. It hadn't happened yet, but the attendant apprehension interfered with her confidence and ability to give herself up to her part. She also had a clearly structural somatic dysfunction of the sixth rib on the right side that interfered with her ability to breathe deeply.

She was seated on the treatment table and I was behind her with my hands on the back of her rib cage to evaluate rib function. This was during the first few minutes of our visit. She seemed to go into a trance as I had my hands on her posterior ribs. Almost immediately a deep voice came from her, saying, "Don't worry about the ribs, my son. That problem will be very easy to correct—or it may correct itself once she has accepted herself into her present reality." Astonished, I wrote this quote down so I wouldn't forget. My mind jumped from astonished to skeptical. I began to make up reasons for her conduct that related to her being a melodramatic actress, or perhaps having multiple-personality disorder, or being totally crazy.

The voice then told me that she had been directed to me because I was open. I translated this as a suggestion that I suspend my skepticism and open myself to what was happening. I was successful at getting my own baggage out of the room. The voice went on and told both of us—for she was able to remember everything after the session—that there were several souls who wanted to communicate with her but she was afraid. Because of this fear, she had been rejecting communication for a long time. I asked the deep voice by what name I could address it. The name given was THEO.

I asked THEO if we had met before. He said no, but he had heard of my healing abilities when I was an apprentice in ancient Greece. He told me that I was well-known and created much jealousy in my elders because of my popularity. He then told me to be careful because they had beheaded me once while I was quite young, and I shouldn't let it happen again. He also told me that, because I was open, I would be used frequently to help souls who were having difficulty getting past certain obstacles. The guides could put into my head what I needed to know, and I would then be able to help these souls get back on course.

I saw this woman once a month for three months. I had no more contact with THEO, but the patient communicated a great deal with her grandfather who had died about twenty years earlier. There seemed to be a lot of advice passed from him to her. As she was able to accept her grandfather's presence without fear, the fainting and dizzy spells ended, as did her fear of their occurrence. (The rib problem had been easily corrected at the end of the first session using an ordinary procedure.) I have not seen this patient since the end of that third session. This singular experience with THEO would have been easy to dismiss were it not coupled with the previously described story of my decapitation in Greece. It was becoming a little more difficult not to accept the experiences at face value.

Next came the clincher.

Bob, Gordon and CAUTHUS

About a week after my encounter with THEO, a forty-two-year-old male named Bob came in from the northeast for a week of treatments. This meant that I would work with him through regular forty-five-minute sessions on Monday, Tuesday, Thursday and Friday of that week.

Monday and Tuesday were such quiet visits that, toward the end of that second session, I asked Bob why he had come to see me. There didn't seem to be any major areas of dysfunction or pain. Bob said that he just wanted to experience the work for which I was, by that time, rather well-known. He said he could afford the luxury.

Thursday he started a SomatoEmotional Release. It involved an old back injury that had occurred while he was a teenage hockey player. He had fallen on the ice. He was mortified. He felt like a fool. No one had pushed or checked him. He was not scrambling for the puck. He was skating up the ice in relative peace when his feet went faster than the rest of his body. It was a Sunday. He was playing hockey for a local dry cleaner's team. His father was watching. He was really embarrassed and angry with himself.

We re-experienced the fall on his tailbone. We released an energy cyst from his lower back via the tailbone route. Along with the energy cyst came the release of embarrassment, mortification, and some self-abuse. He really cussed himself out. He apologized to his father who was very understanding. He finally saw the humor of the whole situation and laughed at himself.

By this time, he was in a deep, pleasant state of relaxation. I asked his Inner Physician if we could talk. The Inner Physician said, "Of course." His Inner Physician's name was Gordon. Gordon said that what we had done would help Bob's self-esteem significantly and that there was nothing else to do that day; the next day, however, we would have a special project to complete.

Bob arrived on Friday for his last in the series of four appointments. He was to fly home that evening. Bob said he'd had a good night. He also said he had gotten in touch with a lot of the self-criticism to which he had been subjecting himself. He thought it was over now. He really had a much nicer feeling about himself and his abilities. I didn't think he would have to go on proving himself so much from now on.

I began the session with a CV-4. Bob went into a state of deep relaxation almost immediately. I asked Gordon if he would care to join us. Gordon responded that he was already present and wanted to introduce someone to me. I indicated I would be most honored to meet anyone Gordon wanted to introduce. Gordon introduced me to CAUTHUS.

CAUTHUS' voice was different—softer, yet more firm. CAUTHUS said, "It is a pleasure to meet you, my son." He told me that it was he who had directed Bob to see me and that he was satisfied with what had been accomplished. I indicated I was surprised that one so evolved as CAUTHUS should be interested in the resolution of residue from a fall on the ice. CAUTHUS became just a little impatient. He let me know that the work we accomplished was much deeper than the fall. He also let me know he was surprised that I was not aware of that. I told CAUTHUS that I simply followed my hands and let whatever happened happen. I tried not to get in the way. CAUTHUS' voice softened again and he said, "Of course, my son. You are open. That is why we can work through you."

I then followed my impulse and asked CAUTHUS if we had known each other before. CAUTHUS told me he had hoped to study healing with me in ancient Greece, but I had been slain by a politicized group of healers before he had the chance. I almost fell off my stool! This was the third time I had been told this same story by the spiritual guides of three different patients who, at least in the here and now, did not know each other. CAUTHUS told me that when you are working out on the edge, there will always be those who try to strike you down.

Three times in three weeks I was told by seemingly independent sources that I had been terminated in ancient Greece by physicians or would-be healers because I was overly precocious and gaining a reputation. All three gave gentle warnings about present-day professional jealousies. All three said they had directed these patients to me because I was "open." It becomes very difficult to discount the authenticity of the information when it comes at you from three separate directions at virtually the same time.

Yes, I do believe that spirit guides are real. And I know deep inside of me that if you go with the flow of things, these guides will tell you precisely what should be done and how to direct your life. It is since the experiences recounted above that I have arrived at the knowledge that spirit guides are real. This is not rational belief; it is gut-level knowledge. Now that I am "open," I have had several experiences with patients in which these guides have played key roles.

Samantha and Her Group of International Guides

At this point, I would like to present a most remarkable clinical case that was more deeply involved with spirit guides than I ever could have imagined. I could easily see why I may have had so many preliminary experiences: They were simply in preparation for this very complex and needy thirty-seven-year-old lady. I will call her Samantha in order to protect her privacy. She is not, however, overly concerned with privacy. She has recounted her experiences to one Somato-Emotional Release class and three Advanced CranioSacral Therapy classes.

Samantha was a successful business executive at the time of her first visit on February 4, 1988. She had been on the professional fast track for about fifteen years prior to this meeting.

She had suffered from endometriosis during her early twenties. This condition creates painful menstrual cycles because uterine-lining tissue is located in places outside the uterus. When a menstrual cycle occurs, there is bleeding from this abnormally located tissue. Blood cysts may form in the lining of the pelvic cavity, on the bowel, or outside the uterus, ovaries, tubes, ligaments, etc.

Samantha stated that she had been successfully treated with some kind of medication but could not remember what it was. She had been on birth control pills on and off for about ten years but had discontinued their use approximately two years prior to this visit. She had not been married nor had she ever been pregnant. She smoked twenty to thirty filtered cigarettes per day and had done so for several years. She claimed only moderate use of alcohol. She had been sexually active, in moderation, for several years.

The reason for this visit was her urgent concern over a lump that had been discovered in her breast. Two days prior to seeing me, she had undergone a mammogram, sonogram and transillumination evaluation that all revealed a suspicious mass in the left breast measuring about 2 centimeters by 0.5 centimeters. This mass was attached to a smaller round mass about 1.1 centimeters in diameter. No masses were noted in the armpit. The right breast showed no suspicious masses, but both breasts had dense fibrocystic tissue with a small proportion of fat.

My own manual examination at this time was done without knowledge of the above test results. I reviewed the reports after I had done my own examination. I recorded the presence of a suspicious mass at eleven o'clock in the left breast, just above the nipple. The mass was attached to the deep side of the skin, which made it very suspicious for malignancy. I estimated its size at about 3 centimeters by 1.5 centimeters with an almost vertical longitudinal axis. I could find no suspicious masses in either of her armpits. Both breasts presented the tissue texture of typical fibrocystic disease.

After my examination and a discussion of my findings and the implications, I asked Samantha why she had chosen to come to me with her problem. She said she had heard of alternative methods of treatment for breast cancer and wanted to know more about them and perhaps give them a try. I suggested that the alternative methods could be a little slow at this stage of the game and might better be used as an adjunct to the surgeon's work. She then told me she was scheduled for a mastectomy on February 19. That gave us two weeks to see what we might be able to do.

I explained the concepts of Therapeutic Imagery and Dialogue to her. She seemed receptive and eager to try this approach. During the CV-4 she became very relaxed. She was able to visualize a quiet beach on which she and I were sunning ourselves. (I wanted to be included in her images right from the start.) We then invited her Inner Physician to join us.

Her Inner Physician seemed eager to accept our invitation. His name was Harold. He told us that the tumor in her breast was malignant and its name was Black Mass. He clearly understood that Black Mass could and would kill Samantha. He suggested that "White Love" in the heart could hold the tumor in abeyance.

Black Mass then spoke to us. He stated that he was tired of living with anger and without love. He would prefer that Samantha die and begin over again with a better attitude. This was a very powerful stance to take at an initial meeting. I negotiated with Black Mass and Samantha. Since the situation was very urgent, I asked if we could please shrink the tumor temporarily and use pain to maintain Samantha's attention and keep her aware of the power of Black Mass. That was agreeable to Black Mass. Harold thought it was a good idea and suggested that the pain should be in the toes of the right foot. Black

Mass agreed. Harold then suggested that I put "loving energy" into Samantha's heart and concentrate with the intention to shrink the tumor. I did my best to follow Harold's suggestions. After about five minutes of concentrated intention, there was a palpable snap in the tumor area. By the time we were finished with the first session, the palpable size of the tumor was reduced by about fifty percent.

When Samantha came back to the here and now, she had no conscious memory of the events that had occurred. She did not remember Harold or Black Mass. I described the session to her and had her feel her tumor. She was astonished to note a significant reduction in the tumor's size and hardness from just an hour before. She was encouraged to hear that I felt quite optimistic about what we would be able to do with this problem.

I asked her about anger and love. She mentioned sexual molestation as a child by both her father and a man named George. We didn't have time to pursue it at that time. She said she thought she had dealt with these problems previously. It didn't seem important to me either. Neither of us felt we could afford to be diverted from focusing on the tumor since surgery was imminent.

Samantha's next visit was eight days later—one week before her surgery. The tumor in the left breast was still about half the size it had been at the beginning of the first visit. I must confess I was probably as excited about this as Samantha.

As I put my hands on her head to begin the session, Samantha went right off into an altered state of consciousness. I asked Harold, her Inner Physician, to join us. He said that he had been helping to clear residual anger and things were looking pretty good.

Then a voice from Samantha spoke with a very powerful British accent. I really had no idea where this came from. I asked who the voice was and it said, "John, have you forgotten me already?" I was totally astonished but tried not to show it. I tried to keep my cool. I explained to this voice that being incarnate and earthbound interfered with memories of past incarnations and spiritual existences. I asked again who the voice was. He said his name was HAWKINS and we had worked together in biological research at Cambridge about two hundred years earlier. He told me that I was always too serious and that he frequently had to take me out of the laboratory to relax. He always took me to a pub where we drank ale and "pinched bottoms."

HAWKINS said he was one of those assigned to Samantha. They knew I would work with them, so they had directed her to me. HAWKINS said she was redeemable and could do a lot of good work if she could be guided past certain obstacles. He was sure we could save her from the cancer.

HAWKINS then suggested that she visualize white blood cells digesting the cancer. He also directed me to put energy directly through the breast. He said he would work with me. I could feel his presence. Harold then suggested that we release the energy of Black Mass into space. We—rather I—could feel the release occur. At the end of the session, the tumor felt about the size of a pea. HAWKINS suggested that I teach Samantha to visualize the white blood cells digesting any cancer remnants. He thought she might not require surgery if we worked fast enough.

Samantha once again awakened with no recall of the session. She felt her lump and immediately realized it was much smaller. I instructed her on the visualization technique of having the white blood cells (they looked like Pac-Man) digest any tumor remnants that were there. She said she would do this visualization daily. When she asked me about her sore right fifth toe, I responded in a very non-committal way. I pondered this HAWKINS fellow.

On February 19, 1988, Samantha underwent a breast biopsy rather than the planned mastectomy because the surgeon had been struck by how much smaller the tumor was now. The tissue that was removed was 1 centimeter in diameter, and it was cancerous. The pathologist did not believe that the tumor was completely excised. There was confusion because the surgeon felt that the mass was totally removed. I can't help but wonder if the surgeon had taken a time-frame study of a malignant tumor in a retrogression/regression stage rather than in an aggressive/invasive stage. I have seldom seen this kind of confusion on reports. All of the other laboratory tests, x-rays, electro-cardiographs, and physical examinations were within the normal ranges and limits.

Samantha's next visit with me was on February 26, just one week after her breast surgery. She was excited because the surgeon was puzzled about the rapid regression in the size of the cancer. Because this was the kind of cancer that often strikes both breasts, she was to go to the surgeon for a biopsy on the other breast just to be sure. That biopsy was scheduled for February 28, just two days later.

Samantha's faith in her own self-healing power was not yet strong enough to resist going through with the second biopsy. She would follow the recommendations of the gynecologist for the right breast biopsy, but she would not have the previously recommended left breast mastectomy with radiation and chemotherapy to follow.

As I put my hands on Samantha's head, she went into her altered consciousness almost immediately. My office assistant was with me now because things had been getting too complicated for me to remember it all. I would not be able to record it accurately and completely on the chart after my hands were free. We asked the Inner Physician to please consult with us. A "Dr. Visor" came on the scene. He told us that anti-cancer white blood cells were his specialty. They were manufactured in the bone marrow. (Samantha told me later, during our conversation at the end of the session, that she knew nothing about white blood cells and where they came from.)

Dr. Visor advised large doses of vitamin B complex and vitamin C from now on. He also said that Samantha should take three large glasses of carrot juice daily as well as supplemental zinc, calcium, chromium and selenium, all in the chelated form. She was also to take the enzymes bromelain and papain.

After this consultation with Dr. Visor, I was inspired to ask who was in charge of the cancer process. This was when "Big C" came forward. A deep, ominous voice came forth from Samantha's very feminine vocal apparatus and told us he was in charge. He informed us that the cancer had come because of the male hormone Danocrine, which Samantha had been given for the endometriosis many years earlier and because of a mineral deficiency. It was now Big C's purpose to draw Samantha's attention to her female side, which had been partially subdued by the Danocrine. He further stated that the minerals advised by Dr. Visor were necessary to restore femininity.

I negotiated with Big C. I told him that he had Samantha's attention and that I would see to it that she knew she would have to get feminine. Negotiation was difficult because Samantha was out of it and could not be brought into the conversation. It felt like we were negotiating her fate without her having any input. I felt like a lawyer must feel trying to avoid the death penalty for a client. In any case, Big C agreed to surrender some of his cancer cells. He gave some up to the white cells and agreed that the molecular structure of some of the malignant cells would be converted back to normal function and status. I was instructed at this time to put energy in through the crown chakra. I was then told to invite Samantha to join us.

This time she responded, although she was still in a deep trance. She was told to visualize Big C putting on a white coat. (He had been wearing a black cape.) Samantha was successful in putting the white coat on Big C. I was then instructed to put energy through the left side of her upper body and breast. When this was done, I was instructed to put energy into the right breast. Big C said he left two cancer cells in the right breast as an insurance policy.

Next, a voice with an Oriental accent was heard. That voice belonged to an entity who introduced himself as LU CHOW PIN. He said he was helping with the energy. LU CHOW PIN was another of the guides assigned to this case along with HAWKINS. While I was getting acquainted with LU CHOW PIN, I simply followed my hands and released the throat, left arm and pubic region to help the hormones. LU CHOW PIN said, "You smart man, blessing all," and left the session. Big C felt confident that Samantha would become a woman as her first priority. He agreed to wear the white coat for awhile. (I assumed this meant he would withhold further malignant activity.)

On February 28, 1988, Samantha went into the hospital for a biopsy of the right breast. No malignancy was found. The biopsy report on the left breast was finalized. It was officially identified as a colloid carcinoma, less than 1 centimeter in diameter. (This offered an official, if not real, end to the confusion of the first biopsy.) It appeared that Samantha had made significant progress toward the resolution of her problem.

Samantha came to see me again on March 2, just one month after her first visit. A lot of water had passed under the bridge for all of us in that one short month. We thought we would be smart and audio-tape the session from start to finish. When we listened to it the first time it was fine, but when we went to listen to it again a week later, all we heard was static. (I mention the audiotape self-destructing because it explains my sketchy notes on this session. I had relied on the audiotape to capture the details. Fortunately, I had two preceptors with me who helped reconstruct the happenings.)

This session was largely conducted by spirit guide LU CHOW PIN. With an inscrutable expression on her face, Samantha spoke again with an Oriental accent. It was most remarkable. LU CHOW PIN recommended that Samantha drink Taheebo tea and make poultices of Taheebo bark to place over the ovaries and breasts for thirty minutes daily. He also advised Samantha to take ginseng. He said it was imperative that she restore her femininity, which had been disturbed by early sexual molestation, by the Danocrine she took for her endometriosis, and by her yang existence in the male business world. LU CHOW PIN also told us that LURIE, a great master, was watching. In addition, Big C's attitude and energy had further softened; he was still a little suspicious and defensive but not as badly. This was a great session. I only wish I had not relied on the audiotape so that my notes would have been more extensive.

Samantha felt wonderful when it was over, but we had to instruct her about everything because she had no idea what happened. She accepted the instructions about Taheebo tea, the poultices and the ginseng. By this time, she was getting used to strange instructions and explanations.

Samantha came for her next session on March 4. I only had to touch her head once. She was in the supine position and assumed the character of LU CHOW PIN immediately. LU CHOW PIN told me that the cancer was all gone. A new character named Luke was to keep the white blood cells active and in good number. Big C was happy. We just did routine hands-on work, got to know LU CHOW PIN better, and had fun.

The next time Samantha visited was on March 31, about four weeks later. The time lapse indicated to me that she was trusting herself and the expertise and power of her protector spiritual guides. I chatted with both LU CHOW PIN and HAWKINS. They both agreed that all was going well. Samantha would now be allowed some grace time to get it together so that she could become a true female. She also had to begin her assigned work, which was to help others to evolve. She was not to continue working in the primitive monetary world of business. I could tell her this, but I was to be gentle and not scare her off. LU CHOW PIN added that the yin (left) side of her body was still confused and that I should put energy through it to help it organize. Also, if she didn't show progress toward the development of her feminine side, she would get pain on the left side. There would be no more cancer unless she rebelled against her new life.

I did not see Samantha again until September 15, 1988. She had gone to New York where her parents lived. While she was there she was persuaded by family and friends to undergo a complete medical workup. They thought it was an act of suicide to refuse a mastectomy, radiation and chemotherapy—even though tests had found no signs of cancer. The fact that she had undergone a lot of criticism and intimidation was apparent. She had more self-doubt than she'd had the first time I saw her. She was also complaining of left arm, shoulder and neck pain. She was afraid this was a cancer recurrence.

During the session Samantha went deeply into her usual trance. The first to introduce himself was EKETAN. He stated that he personally had taken charge of Samantha's case because it was time for her to demonstrate the depth of her faith. He told me to spend as much time with her as seemed advisable because she was at a critical place on her path. He said she had not demonstrated the proper amount of faith when she allowed herself to be persuaded by family and friends to continue fearing the cancer. I was to let her know that she would be fine if she did not divert too much from the path that was being shown her. She would live long enough to do her work, accomplish her growth, and die peacefully when she had fulfilled her assignments.

Then a most remarkable thing occurred. LU CHOW PIN asked to speak with me. EKETAN acceded to this request. He suggested that acupuncture was in order at this time. I asked LU CHOW PIN to tell me what points to needle. He began to name them in Chinese. (I am not competent in locating acupuncture points by Chinese names, but I could recognize the names as being Chinese.) I asked LU CHOW PIN to tell me the points he wanted needled according to the Western system of meridian names and point numbers. He did not know the system. I thought for a minute and asked if he would use Samantha's finger to indicate precisely where he wanted the needles placed. I should mention that all of this dialogue was taking place through Samantha as she assumed her Oriental face and spoke with her unmistakable Oriental accent.

Without much hesitation, Samantha's right index finger pointed to Large Intestine 4, Triple Heater 8, Gallbladder 4, and Liver 8. LU CHOW PIN said, "You will place needles at these points on both sides."

I thought I would try to be helpful and explain the name and number system we use to identify acupuncture points. LU CHOW PIN said this information was of no interest to him. Samantha later denied having any previous knowledge of acupuncture point names and locations.

HAWKINS' wonderful British voice then came through Samantha's throat. He told me I was too serious. He said he wished he could go out for a drink or two with me. I asked him if he could go home with me after work that evening, and he said he could. I asked, "If I drink champagne and you are with me, could you also enjoy it?" He said, "Jolly well would like that." I did go home after work and open a bottle of champagne. I was home alone that evening, so I sat with the champagne and talked to HAWKINS. That night he told me not to worry; he would always be with me to correct my course whenever I might need an adjustment. I just needed to stay open. There I was, drinking champagne and talking to myself!

But let me return to the session with Samantha. EKETAN came back before the session was over. He told me he had a special interest in my work because we had worked together in Egypt. We had been physicians working on the correction of brain disease that caused paralysis. "Disease?" I asked. He asked that I please forgive him; he did not understand all the nuances of the language; he meant "brain injury." He said that all I must do was remain open.

I did not see Samantha and her friends again until March 8, 1989. She stated that the arm, shoulder and neck problem was more persistent. She had gone back on the fast track in business to some extent—not as much as before, but she had made no further moves toward developing a service/teaching career. I thought the pain to be an attention-getter. No structural problem came to my attention. Energy seemed focused and disorganized around the nipple of the left breast. The right breast seemed quiet and organized.

The guide who came forth at this session was CHAMAAS. (I always have them spell their names if they will.) CHAMAAS said he needed help from me with the lower-vibration levels while he worked on the development of her higher-development levels. He requested that I see her weekly for awhile. I agreed to do whatever CHAMAAS suggested, of course. I didn't know what I was doing, but he said I knew on a deeper level because I was doing precisely what he wanted me to do. I am not yet intellectually sure what I was doing in that session. I just thought "lower vibration" in my mind and let my hands do whatever they wanted to do.

Samantha returned on March 19. This time, the guide was JABOOM. He asked me if I had gotten his messages. I said I didn't know. I added that I had felt closed the past week and I apologized. He told me not to expect perfection when working in an earthly body. I was doing fine.

Samantha was amnesic for both the March 9 and March 14 sessions. She had to accept my word that the pain existed to let her know that she was still not giving proper freedom to her femaleness. She must be a woman. She was having trouble letting go of the success and acclaim she had achieved as a business professional. (She was a vice president of a rather large architectural-development firm.)

The next time I saw Samantha on March 23, she said she would not be able to come back to see me again because the insurance wouldn't pay anymore. She would not lie down on the table, but it was a good session. She ventilated a lot of anger about this whole thing. We discussed her "spoiled child syndrome" and her anger at being directed by spirit guides to do something that involved serious life change, risk and sacrifice. She wanted this shoulder pain gone, and she wanted proof that the cancer had not come back. We discussed trust. I told her that if she wanted a mammogram, ultrasound, transillumination, and some blood tests I would order them. She should think about it for a week or so, and then she could go in and get the tests or not; it was her decision. I made it clear that whether or not she got the tests would reflect the level of her trust.

I next saw Samantha on April 14. She had done the tests and they were all negative for any suspicion of cancer. We talked about trust, her resistance to the unfolding of her path, and so on. She had calmed down. The pressure from her family to continually search for cancer was immense. She had a hard time resisting. They couldn't believe she could be cancer-free without having followed the doctors' recommendations. She also got cards from doctors that disclaimed responsibility for her health since she hadn't complied with their recommendations.

We got all of this conversation out of the way, then did a vault hold, a little balancing and a still point. Samantha was once again in her altered state of consciousness. A deep voice came from her. It said, "Greetings, my son. I am BAKANANDA. I have taken charge for the time being. I shall instruct you." He then told me to use my energy to open the glands and ducts of the left breast, thorax, shoulder, and neck. I tried to comply. BAKANANDA said I was doing it just right. I could feel the tissue respond.

I then screwed up my courage and asked BAKANANDA if we could image away the fibrocystic breast disease. He said, "Certainly you can, but it is no concern to those on my plane. That Samantha works on fibrocystic tissue is irrelevant." I took this as a yes. After Samantha came back to the present time and place, we practiced imaging what her breast tissue would look like if it were normal. She agreed to spend perhaps fifteen minutes a day on this work. I hoped that palpable improvement in the texture of her breast tissue would give her what she needed.

Samantha returned to see me on April 27. She went into her altered state almost as soon as she lay down on the table. Once again BAKANANDA came through as the spiritual guide. He advised me that I should now tell Samantha why she had been experiencing so much trouble during the past few months. He told me that Samantha had been a slave in Egypt but had been freed from her enslavement by a group of rebels. She then came to power and enslaved the very people who had liberated her. She was still carrying the burden of that guilt with her. So in addition to embracing her femininity—the rejection of which was due to her enslavement as a female during this lifetime—she also had to let go of her guilt for turning upon her liberators. This had to take place before she could totally uproot the rest of her problem.

BAKANANDA instructed me to energize her spleen and then to open her root chakra (energy center). I did this without difficulty. (Things always seem to go easily when you are doing what you are told to do by a spirit guide.) I let BAKANANDA know how easy it was for me to work when I was guided. He told me it was a pleasure to work with me because I did not question what I was guided to do. I then asked him how I could know when a sense of being guided was authentic. He said I would feel my solar plexus vibrate when it was true. If I was being misled, either by myself or an inferior spirit, I would feel nothing in my solar plexus. So now I'm trying to be aware of my solar plexus when an idea comes to mind.

I then asked BAKANANDA if I could gain some further understanding from him about my life. He said he would help in any way he could. I explained that I felt the teaching of high-purpose intentioned touch was a way of diffusing anger and violence. He told me that he knew about that and what we were doing. He stated that it was part of what needed to be done. I asked him how we could finance the continuation of our work. BAKANANDA said that financing was of no concern on the higher vibratory levels. I told him that we exist on this level, so money has to be a concern to us. Strangely, he responded that he had forgotten we have a M-O-N-E-T-A-R-Y (he spelled the word) system to deal with. It was of no spiritual significance and was just one of those ridiculous things that beings on a lower vibrational plane create in order to make life more difficult and complex. He said they would help as they could, but since it was a system created by incarnate beings, it had to be dealt with primarily on the incarnate level. That answered my question quite clearly: We had to keep on working in the trenches. It may also explain why so many good, spiritually focused projects go bankrupt.

I thanked BAKANANDA for the information he had imparted. I asked if there was anything else he wished to tell me or have me do before we ended this session. He reminded me to gently help Samantha understand the guilt she was carrying for enslaving her liberators back in Egypt.

I gently tried to tell Samantha about the Egyptian experience after she awakened. She could recall no part of our session. She would have to take my word for it if she was to believe it, accept it, and act on it. This required real trust. It didn't help that her left shoulder was still a little painful. The pain suggested to me, however, that her level of trust was not quite what it should be. We discussed this mild deficit in her trust and Samantha agreed to work on it. We then agreed that we would work together about once a month for as long as we felt it to be beneficial.

I next saw Samantha on May 31. She still had some shoulder pain and was mildly upset about it. She wanted some tests done to get to the bottom of this pain. I told her we could get the tests, but I thought we were already at the bottom of the pain and she just didn't want to see it. I did, however, order an arthritis-profile blood test as well as a chem screen (multifaceted screening blood test).

After we drew the blood, Samantha settled down. She had gotten what she needed; now she was ready to work again. She lay on the table and I began balancing her craniosacral system from the vault. She went into a very nice relaxed state. Very suddenly her craniosacral rhythm stopped. The significance detector indicated something was happening.

I asked who was there. A beautiful, loving, feminine voice responded, "It is I, my son, SOUL OF EGYPT." I was surrounded by the most loving, quieting, safe and wonderful atmosphere I had ever experienced. I asked what SOUL OF EGYPT would have me do. This wonderful voice said, "Touch and listen."

Remember the first time you saw the boy or girl of your dreams and fell madly in love? I felt like that. I was tingling from head to toe. I was definitely in love with SOUL OF EGYPT. I asked her for a name by which I could address her. She said SOUL OF EGYPT was all that she wished to tell me.

She then went on to say that she was the soul of Samantha when she was a slave to the pharaoh. She described herself as very beautiful with dark eyes, long black hair and beautiful olive, tanned skin. In return for some political favors, her father had given her to the pharaoh when she was only fifteen years of age. Soon the pharaoh began abusing her sexually. SOUL OF EGYPT described the abuse, which eventually led to the slave's death. I now had to release this energy cyst and its attendant emotion. The release went well. I simply put one hand over the vaginal area (Samantha was wearing street clothes) and the other hand over the left and middle back of the pelvic wall. The release came very easily and was very powerful as an energy vector coming back out of the vagina. I imagined that I could feel the pharaoh's rage and frustration as it exited her body. Maybe I did feel it; I'm not sure of these things anymore.

SOUL OF EGYPT then thanked me for being so helpful. She bade me farewell and I could feel the wonderful vibrations gently and slowly leave the room. There I sat, with my hands on Samantha's pelvis, almost totally in shock. I went back up to Samantha's head, collected my wits, and brought her back to the present.

As usual, she remembered nothing. As I described SOUL OF EGYPT, Samantha's eyes shined like I had never seen them shine before. She softened and seemed to suddenly trust. I told her about her experiences with the pharaoh and her death. I tried to help her accept what had happened. I described how the pharaoh's energies were released from her body. She told me this felt like another part of the reason she was denying her femininity in this lifetime.

It was a good session with good closure. When I think about SOUL OF EGYPT, I still feel totally in awe and somewhat like a smitten teenager.

I called Samantha a couple of days later to let her know that her laboratory results were normal. For the first time, she seemed disinterested. She said she knew they were normal and would look forward to seeing me in three or four weeks.

My last visit with Samantha before writing this account of our experiences together occurred on June 28, 1989. She was in good spirits that day. She no longer seemed worried about the presence of cancer in her body. We chatted a little while as I began working with her craniosacral system. The urgency to go into deep trance seemed less dominant. After a few minutes I asked whether there was anyone who would like to speak with us today. Within a minute or so after my inquiry, Samantha was deep into her altered state of consciousness. A gentle feminine voice came from Samantha. The voice informed us that her name was EUJUTA and that SOUL OF EGYPT sent her love. EUJUTA then told me that I must continue to work with Samantha until her heart chakra (energy center) remained open and flowing. I asked how often that should be, and she told me about once a month should be fine.

Next, EUJUTA wanted to give us some information regarding physical sex and spiritual love. She stated that physical sex with love in the proper setting promoted spiritual connection between the participants. This spiritual union promoted unconditional love and thus spiritual evolution. Physical sex without high spiritual meaning was for lust. Lust obstructs the path toward spiritual advancement.

Monogamy on the physical plane is a human creation of little spiritual importance, except that it may get in the way of the union of several spirits who may be ready to connect. We must know that physical sex is not required for spiritual connection. It does, however, facilitate spiritual connection when the physical sex is done with good intent rather than for reasons of lust.

With these comments, EUJUTA departed the session. The heart chakra (energy center) was open. Since Samantha was a single woman, I suspected that EUJUTA'S comments about spiritual love and its relationship to physical sex were meant to clarify some confusion in Samantha's mind.

IM

Gary was a forty-one-year-old male who first came to us during the summer of 1988. I did not see him during that time. He was treated by one of the other osteopathic physicians here at The Upledger Institute HealthPlex clinic.

The man returned for a week of treatments in November 1988. I did one session with him at that time. During this session he re-experienced and went through the SomatoEmotional Release of his tonsillectomy and then his birth trauma.

In June of 1989 Gary returned for another week of treatments. This time I had four sessions with him. During the first session I worked toward the release of a chronic left arm and shoulder pain syndrome. During the second session his voice changed and he spoke to me as an individual who called himself IM. IM told me that there was a group of scientists who were close to perfecting a "time suspension" machine. This machine was capable of suspending the passage of time for a given individual. Gary was to see that this was used for good and not for wrongful purposes. Gary was to discuss this with Mr. Gorbachev of the Soviet Union. Later, at the end of this session, I found out that Gary and Gorbachev, along with some others, were indeed to have a meeting in the late summer of 1989. Gary's memory regarding the content of this session was sketchy when he returned to full consciousness.

I had two more sessions with Gary that week. We did some rather routine upper thoracic and cervical structural work. IM returned during both of these sessions with information for me. He stated that he was the messenger. He did not understand the meaning of what he was about to share, but I was to think about it, as it would ultimately be very important in my own work. IM then proceeded to describe a cylinder made of transparent Lucite material mounted in a gyro-type machine. Within this cylinder was what I interpreted to be the double helix of DNA. IM didn't know what it was; he could only describe it. He also told me that it had to do with the work we were doing against the spread of violence. He could tell me no more.

SARAH

I can't end this chapter without sharing one more experience that I had with another female patient. Her guide, SARAH, was communicating with me freely and offering advice and wisdom throughout the session. I finally asked SARAH if there was anything else she would like me to do before ending the session. SARAH was quiet for a minute and then said, "No, I think we've done what was necessary." I thanked her and asked if it was okay if I popped the seventh cervical vertebra on the patient's right side. SARAH said, "Go ahead if you think you should, but wait a minute until I get out of here." I waited a few seconds. I'm sure I felt an energy change. Then I used a direct thrust on the seventh vertebra. The patient awakened within seconds after the pop. She exclaimed, "You've popped my neck."

Channeling Postscript

These are some of the more outstanding experiences I have had while working with patients. It is, of course, possible to dismiss these experiences as nonconscious parts of the psyche making their presence known, or perhaps as manifestations of "multi-personality disorder," or even as psychotic episodes. You can also make a case for either the patient or me being the psychotic one. But if you are there, it isn't quite so easy to write them off as non-spiritual experiences. In the previous chapter, which describes my personal experiences, it is made clear that I was a firm skeptic some years ago. Now I am quite open and leaning toward the idea that there are spirit guides who offer a lot of very good wisdom to those of us who will accept it. I am sure that I accepted a lot of wise advice for many years, even while I thought I was a skeptic.

The events I have described did occur. Most often there was a preceptor in the room with us, so there is verification of the events described. There were several other such experiences. Those I have described here are exemplary.

Some time later I had one more visit with Samantha. I had a preceptor named Harvey with me. To the best of our recollection, the dialogue content is paraphrased below. Neither of us will ever forget this experience.

Samantha came into the session in a very positive mood. She stated that she was still working as a business professional and was participating as one of the sponsors in an "energy healing" seminar that weekend. She was elated about this opportunity.

She had only one concern about her body at the time of this visit. There was a small but palpable lump in her left armpit. She pointed it out to me; it was definitely there. It was about the size of a pea. I think that I was more concerned than she was because I put on my traditional physician's hat immediately and started to worry that this lump might be a metastatic tumor that had spread from her left breast, which was the site of her original malignancy.

I tuned into her craniosacral rhythm with a vault hold. Harvey sat near her head as a silent observer. She relaxed easily. Within just a few minutes she was deep in a relaxed, trancelike state. I asked very gently and quietly if there was anyone there who would advise and help us during the session that day. Her face sort of screwed up around her mouth and her lips pursed. A rather deep voice said, "There are two." I misunderstood and thought that I was encountering an entity named Too or Tuo. I enquired about the spelling. The voice from Samantha became a little impatient-sounding and said, "There are two today." There was a little interchange about 'two,' 'too' and 'Tuo' and an apology on my part, and then the voice from Samantha introduced itself as JAMOOZE.

I commented on the beauty and uniqueness of the names of the guides I had encountered during my work with Samantha. JAMOOZE explained that the names were created for our benefit by those on his plane because we seemed to need names as we worked. On his plane they had no use for names. This was why they were sometimes slow to respond when we asked for a given entity by name. JAMOOZE said that all entities on higher planes know one another by vibration. He then said that HAWKINS sent me his love.

JAMOOZE informed me that all was going well with Samantha. He said that the "hardness" in the breast where the surgical biopsy had been done was breaking up and dissolving. I asked about the lump that Samantha had pointed out to me. He said, "You mean in the pit arm?" I didn't understand pit arm. He repeated pit arm a little impatiently, and I finally realized what he meant. I said, "Oh, you mean the armpit?" He just mumbled something about "pit arm, armpit, what is the difference?"

JAMOOZE directed me to open the channel between the root and the crown chakras through the vertical core of her body. He then instructed me to use Harvey's hands in addition to my own. He said that Harvey was not there by accident; his connection was desired.

Harvey was to open the lower body core with one hand and do the spleen with the other. I used one hand on the crown chakra and then, at JAMOOZE'S instruction, I placed one finger on the lump in Samantha's "pit arm." JAMOOZE told us to connect the upper and lower body by opening the core. At the same time, Harvey was to energize the spleen while I dissolved the lump. In a matter of a few minutes, it all worked just as JAMOOZE said it would.

Samantha's face went all soft and radiant. You could feel the love in the air. You could almost cut it with a knife it was so prominent. A beautiful voice issued forth from Samantha's new face. The voice said, "I am ILNA. I come to bring love and gentleness to this healing." ILNA then told me that Samantha was doing extremely well. All I had to do from now on was to be sure that the heart chakra remained open. She said, "It is necessary that it remain open so that love can flow freely in and out. There can be no disease when the heart chakra is open and love flows freely." ILNA then made a flat statement that allowed for no discussion or argument. She said, "There is no disease without conflict." I repeated it three or four times to be sure I understood correctly. ILNA repeated again after each of my responses, "Yes, my son, it is true. There is no disease without conflict." I finally understood the broad application of this statement.

A statement then came from ILNA that took me totally by surprise. She said, "Print twice as many copies of your book as you think you should. It will be very much in demand." I asked her what book she meant. She said the book I was just finishing. Then she told me they were all pleased that I had followed their suggestion. I asked what suggestion that was. ILNA said they had told me about a year before to begin writing this book. I had objected a little, but when they gave me the message to sit down and start writing, I did, and they were pleased.

I then said that, as long as we were on the topic of the book, perhaps she could help with a question that had come up in discussion. It involved the possible loss of credibility I might suffer by putting into print the rather detailed descriptions of some of the incredible experiences in which I have been privileged to participate. We were just beginning to discuss the possibility of editing out some of the more far-out descriptions for fear of losing some of our developing support, when ILNA said simply, "Do not edit. Stand on your feet. Put your head up. And tell the truth." There wasn't much room for doubt about her statement. Everything I have written is the truth to the best of my ability to remember and know; it should not be edited. ILNA then went on to say that those who were close to me who advised editing did not know that the time was right nor understand the importance of the message. Some would have difficulty with what I presented. She hoped they would be challenged to evolve and grow to new levels of advancement, but if they weren't, that was their choice. ILNA then said, "Be at peace, my son. We are pleased." She left.

Samantha slowly came back to the here and now. I asked her to find the lump in her left armpit (or was it pit arm?). She couldn't find it and was very pleased.

I asked her if she knew I had just finished the manuscript of a new book. She said she did not. Then she thought for a minute and said that she had possibly heard something about me beginning a new book about a year before, but she wasn't sure.

So, my friends, the manuscript for the book you hold in your hands remained uncut. I have complete trust in my guides.

Chapter Seven

Some Additional Case Histories

In this chapter I would like to present a sampling of case histories I have collected over the years since I began applying CranioSacral Therapy as a therapeutic modality.

Case of Long-Standing Cephalgia (Head Pain) Treated by CranioSacral Therapy

The patient—a thirty-six-year-old, well-developed, well-nourished Caucasian female—came to the office on July 7, 1974. She was unable to walk due to severe pain in the head and dizziness. She complained of numbness of the tongue and the left arm. She also complained of a loss of vision in the left eye. The visual disturbance had been episodic in nature for many years. She stated that the whole right side of her head was extremely painful. She had endured these headaches three or four times a week for as long she could remember. She brought medical records with her from a local neurologist. These records were non-contributory except to rule out a CNS (central nervous system) lesion and/or tumor. The patient stated she had been to at least twenty doctors over the past fifteen to twenty years. She had received some temporary help after chiropractic treatment; however, the relief usually lasted only a few hours. Headaches were almost always accompanied by nausea and vomiting. Unfortunately this patient did not receive any relief from standard migraine medications. Her blood pressure was normal at 110/70. Her lungs were clear of any abnormal sounds and her heart sounds were normal.

Since the patient was in such a distressed condition, further routine physical examination was deferred at the time of the first visit. Examination of the cervical spine and paravertebral musculature revealed muscle splinting on the right side. There was a restriction of the motion of the neck due to increasing pain in the head.

Compression of the fourth ventricle was performed. This procedure gave the patient about 50 percent relief from the headache. I then proceeded to examine the cranial bones and their function. Examination revealed a rather marked side-bending lesion to the right. This lesion corrected, assisted by the patient's own respiratory mechanism. There was also lesioning of the temporal-parietal and temporal-occipital sutures on the right side. These lesions were corrected by directing the fluid from the opposite side.

The patient stated that the headache was relieved almost immediately following correction of the side-bending lesion of the sphenobasilar symphysis. She became extremely sleepy. Her husband was instructed to put her to bed and let her sleep as long as she wished.

The patient was seen again five days later. She stated that she had been very tired and had experienced some nausea the day following the initial treatment. The neck stiffness had persisted for two days. The severe headache had not returned since the time of the first visit. Examination of the cranial vault revealed no discernible cranial lesion patterns at this time, and examination of the sacral mechanism revealed it to be functioning well. Her blood pressure was 110/66. The problem in the cervical area seemed to have dissipated rather well. There was good motion in the cervical spine. No specific osteopathic paravertebral lesions were noted. The musculature seemed to be of normal tonus and was equal bilaterally (on both sides).

The patient was seen a month later (five weeks after the first treatment). She had suffered no headaches in the interim. She stated that this was the first time in her life she had gone more than three days without a severe headache. Examination of the cranium revealed no significant cranial lesion pattern. There was an atlanto-occipital lesion (posterior occiput) on the right. This was corrected using a thrusting manipulative procedure.

This patient was last seen three months after that visit, which represents a period of more than four months. Examination of the craniosacral mechanism was non-contributory. The patient stated that she had had no return of headaches since the day following the first visit. It is felt that this patient probably suffered the sphenobasilar symphysis lesion early in life (possibly at the time of birth). This lesion was the probable cause of the headaches.

CranioSacral Therapy: The Case of Olivier Scheps

I first saw Olivier Scheps, a Belgian-born male, as part of a demonstration on CranioSacral Therapy held in Nice, France, in July 1979.

Olivier, who was born on November 25, 1975, had been diagnosed as having cerebral palsy when he was fifteen months old. At the age of three and a half, after intensive conventional therapy, he could not walk, was not toilet-trained, and suffered from strabismus (crossed eyes) and nystagmus (spasmodic motion of the eyeball). He was unable to chew or swallow correctly and had never eaten solid food.

Physical Development

Olivier's mother reported that his APGAR score had been within normal bounds. (AGPAR is an evaluation of physiological function done soon after obstetrical delivery.) At five days of age, however, while still hospitalized, he had suffered unexplained vomiting, diarrhea and hypothermia (low body temperature). He also would lapse into long periods of comalike sleep, with no movement in the facial or eye muscles.

At fifteen months of age, Olivier would only lie where he was put. After four months of physiotherapy he was able to turn on one side. He later was treated specifically for cerebral palsy by Dr. Bobath of London and Dr. Voyta of West Germany. At three years of age he began crawling in a sideways fashion, rather like a crab. He pulled his right side along using his left arm and leg. His spasticity was so great that he was unable to sit alone.

Olivier's Perception

Olivier's mother reported that he enjoyed listening to music and was talking in complete sentences at one year of age. At fifteen months he expressed his frustration with his physical condition by telling his mother he wanted to run in the garden.

He eventually conceptualized his situation by referring to two persons: "B," the good boy who could do everything; and the "gros batard," the incompetent boy who could do nothing. He also described a "man knocking" inside his head at the point of the right temporal-parietal suture. He often was closed and withdrawn, and he allowed his mother to do everything for him because he didn't wish to move.

CranioSacral Therapy

Olivier's response to CranioSacral Therapy was so remarkable that experts observing his treatments in Nice suspected that twins—one normal and one with cerebral palsy—were being used in the demonstrations.

After his first fifteen- to thirty-minute treatment, Olivier insisted on trying to walk on his own. After the second treatment, he began indicating for the first time when he needed to go to the toilet. After the third day of treatment, he was feeding himself solids.

During the third treatment I noted a release of the left coronal suture where it overlays the motor cortex. After this Olivier's spasticity abated. The next day Olivier walked into the room holding only his mother's hand.

Olivier's behavior changed as dramatically as his physical condition. He was very proud of his accomplishments and declared his new-found independence and initiative. He became an active, busy child, able to handle motor skills such as doing puzzles and building vertical constructions.

Olivier was brought to the United States in late September 1979 for continuing therapy with me. Toward the end of these treatments, a release was noted at the right temporal-parietal suture—the point where he had indicated the knocking. Thirty seconds later Olivier was in deep sleep.

After this session Olivier indicated that the "man knocking" had left, as had the pain he had experienced in his knee, feet, elbow and wrist. In addition, he said that both "B" and "gros batard" were "on holiday." He told his mother that he thought the doctor had completed his work, and he commented repeatedly on how well he felt.

For a four-year-old child, Olivier's behavior during CranioSacral Therapy was remarkable. He willingly remained relaxed and immobile during the half-hour procedures, and his enjoyment of the therapy and the therapists was obvious. He spent much of the time trying to teach the staff French. He also played some sophisticated verbal jokes in the process, such as trying to teach me that his nose was not a "nez" but a "zi-zi."

Except for the consequences of his muscular atrophy, Olivier's motor skills are now developing normally. He can walk well and jump and ride a tricycle.

I see Olivier every few years. He is doing well, and when I last spoke with him by telephone he was about to enter law school in Brussels, Belgium.

CranioSacral Therapy and Animals

I have frequently been asked whether CranioSacral Therapy is effective on animals. I'm sure that it is, although I can only speak from my own experience using it on dogs. I feel that an experience with our then seven-month-old Bichon Frise, Maddie, is worth sharing because I believe it tested the limit of CranioSacral Therapy's efficacy and its potential in the animal kingdom.

We were fortunate to obtain Maddie from a friend, Judith Sullivan, when her Bichon, Snowflake, had her litter. Maddie weighed about eleven pounds, was pure white, cute as a button, and we loved her dearly.

On Sunday evening, November 11, 1986, Maddie was out in our screened-in pool area. There were many plants on either end of the enclosure. We often had frogs and lizards inside this area, and in three years had seen three snakes.

Maddie came into the house and began acting curiously. She was restless and fearful, was running around the living room, and started to cry and yelp. The left flue (at the mouth) was quite swollen and red. I thought she must have been bitten by a lizard or snake. She then had a mild seizure, which was followed by a rapidly deepening limp and stuporous stare. We called the emergency veterinary clinic and described the situation. The doctor felt from the description that Maddie had probably bitten a poisonous toad on the back. He explained that the poison was neurotoxic and could be deadly, so we had better get her to the clinic right away. While I was on the phone, Maddie vomited and had diarrhea. I washed out her mouth to get rid of any excess and unabsorbed poison. By this time her gums were very white as were her flues and the insides of her ears.

We headed quickly to the vet clinic. My wife drove and I held Maddie. Maddie got progressively more limp and non-arousable. She also showed very rapid, shallow breathing, as well as a rapid and faintly palpable heartbeat. About halfway to the clinic (a thirty-minute drive) I decided to do some cranial work. Her head was extremely extended and contracted. I just thought hard about membrane relaxation and expansion. I began to get a cranial rhythm, which increased in amplitude and improved in its relaxed quality very quickly. As these craniosacral system changes occurred, her breathing slowed and seemed more powerful, and I could feel energy beginning to fill her body. Within a few minutes it was clear that she was not going to die in my arms.

When we got her to the vet clinic she was rousable and stable. It suggests that CranioSacral Therapy might be a good emerging technique to use for a toxic animal.

In the Nick of Time

In the autumn of 1996, I completed five intense CranioSacral Therapy sessions with a two-year-old boy who had suffered from intractable seizures since birth. During our week of single sessions, it appeared to me that the origin of the seizures was in the left temporal lobe. The father confirmed that a PET scan had suggested that the left temporal lobe was indeed the source of the trouble.

Our work suggested that a diagonal application of forceps used in haste during childbirth because of fetal distress was the cause of a rather marked distortion in the structure and function of the child's cranial vault. It was also clear that the umbilical cord was around the neck at delivery and the mandible was severely compressed posteriorly. This latter observation suggested a face-anterior (star gazer) delivery position of the fetal head with compression not only on the mandible but on the nose and glabella by the maternal pubic region.

All of these findings were confirmed by the father, who was present at the delivery. There was also a torsion of the dural tube, which I presume was most likely secondary to a hard pull by the forceps to deliver this distressed baby in a hurry. (His heart rate had slowed below normal.)

This child cried and fought hard during our treatment session until I was able to release the temporal bones laterally, correct the severe cranial vault distortion, and decompress the forehead, face and mandible. After that he slept through the treatment process.

He also had several seizure episodes during the treatments. These seizures told me that I was working in the right place: the temporal region and the tentorium cerebelli. At first, traction on the left ear and/or on the left tentorium increased seizure activity. Then, as the strain pattern improved, the seizures began to lessen in intensity. My prognosis for this child is excellent.

Here is the scary part. This child had been on anti-seizure medications since birth. The medications had not been effective in any combination or individually. As a result, the pressure was on to have surgical intervention to stop the seizures. I couldn't believe my ears when the father told me that his son was one day away from surgery to remove the left temporal lobe.

The temporal lobes are where the hippocampus resides. The hippocampus is the triage officer in charge of what gets remembered and where that memory is stored. The ears hear through the temporal lobes. Plus, both the planum temporale and limbic system are located in large part in the temporal lobes. The planum temporale enables us to put our thoughts into words, phrases and sentences that are intelligible to other people. And the limbic system is associated with autonomic functions and certain emotions and behaviors. So removal of one temporal lobe would have to reduce feelings, etc.

What all this means is that removal of the temporal lobe would turn this child into a non-feeling, robotic type of individual—all because the doctors couldn't figure out how to ease the seizures.

During the week we worked together, this young child began speaking and putting together sounds more effectively. I would be willing to make a sizeable wager that a skilled practitioner trained in CranioSacral Therapy could have corrected this child's problems with an hour or less of treatment in the first day or two of his life. Had this been done, perhaps all the anguish, medication, delayed development, etc., might have been avoided.

When the Immune System Attacks the Liver, Find Out Why

I saw Edith, a seventy-year-old woman, only once. She came to see me on June 6, 2000, bringing with her a diagnosis of autoimmune disease of the liver. This diagnosis was made at the Mayo Clinic in Rochester, Minnesota. Her blood chemistry reports were consistent with significant liver disease. The autoimmune diagnosis was made by biopsy of the liver.

I evaluated her using the usual CranioSacral Therapy approach. I was drawn to her liver and secondarily to her lower throat in the region of the thymus gland. The vitality of her craniosacral system was markedly reduced.

I blended with her and, as we became one, I was moved to talk to her immune system cells. Should these cells be willing to dialogue with me, perhaps I could find out why they were attacking the liver cells. First I asked Edith whether she would allow her immune system components to speak with me using her vocal apparatus. She agreed. As is so often the case she was now deep in an altered state of consciousness.

I asked the thymus gland if it would be willing to speak with me. Edith's voice answered yes quite enthusiastically. I asked the thymus gland if it knew about the immune cells destroying the liver cells. It answered yes again, and added that these were abnormal liver cells that were being destroyed. The attacking immune cells were macrophages working under thymus gland's direction. I asked thymus gland if it knew what happened to the liver cells to make them abnormal. Once again, the answer was yes. The explanation given was as follows.

About four years earlier, Edith had received x-ray therapy following the removal of some malignant growths from her colon. The x-ray exposure had changed the DNA of some of the liver cells. These changed cells had divided and produced more cells that were abnormal. This had been going on for awhile before thymus gland received information about the existence and multiplication of these abnormal/changed liver cells. Now it was the immune system's job to clear all abnormal cells from the liver.

Clearly this "autoimmune" disease of the liver was the immune system's effort at restoring the liver to health. If one simply looked at liver function tests and then studied the biopsy materials under the microscope, it would certainly seem to be autoimmune disease. Taken from this view at this particular time, it appeared that the macrophage cells of the immune system were destroying "healthy" liver cells. The microscope did not yet show that the liver cells being destroyed were dysfunctional.

I applauded the thymus gland and the whole immune system for removing these abnormal liver cells in order to protect the normal part of the liver from invasion. Blood samples taken did, in fact, indicate elevated levels of liver enzymes. These enzymes escape into the blood when liver cells are being damaged or destroyed. Also, bilirubin levels in the blood were elevated. Bilirubin is one of the by-products of the normal degradation of red blood cells. This degradation produces hemoglobin, which then further degrades to bilirubin among other things. These abnormal blood tests were what prompted the liver biopsy.

I let thymus know that, although what it was doing was correct and necessary, we should do something about constructing new and normal liver cells to take the place of the abnormal ones that were being destroyed. Thymus agreed. I suggested that we might be able to recruit some stem cells from the bone marrow to go to the liver and develop new and normal liver cells. Thymus agreed again. I asked thymus if we could communicate with the sternum's (breast bone) marrow regarding our plan. Thymus told me to go ahead.

I asked the sternal marrow if it would speak with me. The answer was yes. I explained the situation thus far and requested that sternal marrow send stem cells to the liver to contract liver cells and restore normal function. During this request I had my hand on the sternum. I could feel energetic activity under my hand as sternal marrow agreed to honor my request. I then moved my hand to the liver. In less than a minute I could feel a new and different activity in the liver. I assumed that this new energy represented the stem cells in action. Stem cells have the capability of creating new and compatible cells in almost any tissue they visit. The bone marrow is like a holding residence for these stem cells; there they await instructions to go to various needy organs and/or tissues. This done, I did some balancing CranioSacral Therapy.

Edith came back to the here and now with full memory and awareness of what we had done. She had two follow-up sessions with one of our in-house therapists, Francine, who administered general Cranio-Sacral Therapy. Francine confirmed the therapeutic dialogue with the immune system and the stem cells, and she congratulated the liver.

Blood tests done eleven days after Edith's last treatment with Francine showed significant improvement in liver function. Edith reported that she felt much more energetic and vital. Repeat liver tests were done on September 29, 2000, and were all within normal limits. These latter tests were done less than three months after her treatments with us.

Had we not established dialogue and rapport with Edith's immune system and bone marrow stem cells, she would have been treated with immunosuppressant drugs to stop the macrophages from "attacking" the liver. The abnormal liver cells would probably have continued to multiply, perhaps resulting in liver failure or possibly liver cancer.

It seems quite worthwhile for healthcare professionals to try something as harmless as dialoguing with systems, organs, tissues, etc. Of course, it requires an ego sacrifice on their part and an honoring of the possibility that cells have consciousness too.

Chapter Eight

Intensive Programs
at The Upledger Institute

The Upledger Institute (UI) HealthPlex Clinical Services

At The Upledger Institute we train experienced medical professionals as well as select lay personnel in CranioSacral Therapy, Somato-Emotional Release and related therapies. Our Upledger Institute HealthPlex Clinical Services offers private sessions as well as one- and two-week outpatient intensive therapy programs developed to meet special needs. Each intensive program is limited to a small number of participants and is conducted by a specially selected team of CranioSacral Therapists and other clinicians working together to alleviate the specific health concerns of each individual.

The health conditions these programs address cover a wide range of problems that CranioSacral Therapy has been useful in treating. They include: migraine headaches, traumatic brain and spinal cord injuries, chronic neck and back pain, motor-coordination impairments, stress and tension-related problems, central nervous system disorders, temporomandibular joint dysfunction, orthopedic problems, chronic fatigue, scoliosis, neurovascular disorders, immune disorders, infantile disorders, colic, post-traumatic stress disorder, autism, post-surgical dysfunction, learning disabilities of all types, fibromyalgia, and other connective-tissue disorders.

These programs involve whatever modalities are found to be appropriate, using CranioSacral Therapy as the base. Clients work with individual and multiple CranioSacral Therapy facilitators. They also participate in group support sessions with other attending clients. Husbands, wives, parents and other caregivers are invited to participate in ShareCare® workshops. These are one-day seminars that give individuals and their caregivers, families, friends and other interested persons a better understanding of the craniosacral system and CranioSacral Therapy in particular. ShareCare covers the basic anatomy and physiology of the system along with the research and development of the therapy. Participants also are instructed in a few basic therapy techniques they can safely use to reduce stress and relieve pain.

UI HealthPlex publishes the *UpClose* newsletter for practitioners, clients and interested readers to help them keep in touch with therapeutic developments, research projects, etc. Most of the stories that follow are excerpted from *UpClose* newsletters over the years. The exception is the last story, which is from a detailed journal kept by the mother of a boy who was taking part in an intensive program. It gives an excellent account of what the intensive programs are actually like.

CranioSacral Therapy Helps Migraines and More

April 1998—In 1988, when Lisa suffered a stroke due to an aneurysm that burst in her brain, she was left with loss of sensation in her right leg, restricted motion in her right arm, and debilitating migraine headaches. Her husband needed to cope not only with his wife's illness but with a healthcare system that had undergone radical change.

"I had to deal with Lisa's condition not as a doctor, but as a spouse and caregiver," husband Barry, a psychiatrist, recalls. "The physicians didn't want to talk to us. They didn't want to discuss emotion-laden issues, like can she walk, talk or drive. What they don't see is that their words shape the way patients look at the future and they can take away hope."

Lisa's recovery was interrupted by two surgeries in 1992. Doctors also discovered that she had developed hepatitis as a result of the medications. Just months later, Hurricane Andrew destroyed their home, their son's house, and the hospital where Barry worked.

They regrouped. Lisa was involved in another rehabilitation program near their new home in Aventura when three different therapists recommended that she come to the UI HealthPlex to seek relief of migraine headaches she had suffered since childhood.

"When we met Dr. Upledger, we felt good about him," Barry recalls. "We liked the fact that he was down-to-earth and we weren't given a lot of hype about CranioSacral Therapy."

Not only did Lisa's headaches diminish within five sessions, but she regained feeling in her right leg that was lost after the stroke. The feeling and freedom of movement in her right arm increased and her vision improved.

Encouraged that she could make more progress, Lisa registered for UI's intensive therapy program and entered a new, positive healthcare environment.

CranioSacral Therapy Adds the Missing Piece to Stroke Rehab

November 1998—When Larry came to a South Florida hospital in October 1996 for a medical test, he never imagined that it would be a week before he could leave. During the test Larry suffered a stroke that affected his speech and the use of his right arm.

Speech and occupational therapy and cardiac rehabilitation were recommended to help him recover. But when Larry wasn't making gains at the rate he expected, his wife suggested he see her therapist, Dr. John Upledger, and try CranioSacral Therapy.

After the first session, Larry's wife and daughter noticed improvement in his speech. But what happened after the second session surprised everyone, including Larry. Without thinking about it, he picked up a pen and signed a check, something he had been unable to do. Comparing that signature with the one on his driver's license, Larry was pleased to find that the two matched.

Larry's progress continued and he went ahead with planned cardiac surgery. During each of two operations, he suffered subsequent strokes.

But CranioSacral Therapy helped him rebound and enabled him to return to work as a salesman for a Rhode Island-based jewelry company in May 1997. He continued to work until his retirement four months later.

When his friends ask about his impressive recovery, Larry tells them, "Faith in God first, doctors who took good care of me, and good treatment from Dr. Upledger."

A fourth stroke last November during gallbladder surgery brought Larry back for a few more CranioSacral Therapy sessions. "I'm as good as I can get," he says today.

Multiple Sclerosis Symptoms Bring Woman to HealthPlex

October 1996—This fall brings new promise for Debbie Sibley of Virginia. She's looking forward to bicycle rides with her kids and returning to work as a special education teacher.

For the past two years, Debbie's life has been disrupted by surgeries, doctors' visits and, mostly, pain. It started with complications from a series of serious surgeries that kept her in the hospital for forty-five days—six in intensive care. The surgery was repeated less than a year later. This time, she was out of work for five months.

Just when Debbie was beginning to feel better, she noticed severe pain in her left leg. She thought she had a slipped disc, but surgery was not an option for her. An orthopedist recommended physical therapy; other doctors suggested medication. The symptoms continued and were diagnosed as degenerative disc disease. One doctor ordered injections to ease the pain. But Debbie didn't want to depend on drugs, so she saw a different doctor. A spinal tap was being considered.

"They started tossing around the diagnosis of multiple sclerosis (MS) and I called The Upledger Institute in a panic," Debbie recalls. "I had to do something. The symptoms were so bad."

Debbie came to The Upledger Institute HealthPlex clinic this summer for the two-week intensive program. "I don't remember the last time I felt this good," Debbie says. One noticeable difference is that her balance is better. Instability had caused her to stop bike riding. After one week in the program, Debbie was able to sleep through the night without being awakened by pain. At the same time, she began taking the stairs to the second floor treatment facility—on the first day of the program she had barely been able to walk down the hall.

In addition to relieving her symptoms, the intensive program gave her peace of mind, a sense of well-being and hopefulness, Debbie says. She plans to continue CranioSacral Therapy back home in Virginia. And she's going to ride her bike whenever she can.

Pilot Keeps Dream Alive

October 1997—Ken's dream is to fly again one day. As a member of the Air National Guard and a commercial pilot, he felt a special joy in flying. But that feeling was taken away in June 1993 when his F-15 fighter crashed outside New Orleans.

The thirty-three-year-old Louisiana native has come a long way since the accident that resulted in a significant head injury. Ken was in a coma for thirty-two days.

After years under the care of the Department of Veterans Affairs, he had made a good recovery and enjoyed a great deal of independence. But he still didn't feel like the man he was before the accident— he was not nearly ready to return to flying.

With his dream still in sight, he sought out other therapies that would continue his progress. He found CranioSacral Therapy and had weekly sessions with Sue Guynes, P.T., in New Orleans. Guynes recommended the intensive therapy program at the UI HealthPlex.

But the question of how much further Ken could go seemed to be in the hands of a VA physician. Would the VA pay for this therapy?

"The VA doctor had heard about UI," Ken says. "But he felt it wasn't worth his time to consider it."

In the end, however, Ken believes it was his father's tenacity in pushing through the paperwork that got the doctors to "give him a break" and allow him to come to the UI HealthPlex.

"For me it's been a Godsend. My speech has improved so very

much, and my mind. And my hand—it used to shake," Ken says. "These are minute details, but they mean a lot to me."

As an example of the improvements that occurred during the intensive program, Ken cites his morning routine of devotional reading aloud. "My dad heard me the other day and he really noticed a difference. It used to take me more time, but now I can read two or three sentences in a row," Ken says.

His dream of flying is once again alive and well.

Child Rebounds From Pediatric Strokes

April 1998—Eliane, two years old, arrives for a day of therapy dressed in yellow and looking like a buttercup. It's the second intensive therapy program at UI HealthPlex that the little girl from Cornwall, Ontario, has attended after suffering a shower of strokes in June 1997.

"CranioSacral Therapy gave her a new lease on life," Eliane's mother, Ginette, says. "There is no question in my mind that she would not be where she is today without it."

Now Eliane is on the brink of crawling, eats soft foods, and reacts with delight as her mother crosses the room—a stark contrast to the child who hospital workers predicted would be blind and wheelchair-bound.

Ginette explains that the strokes produced seizures in Eliane, who was hospitalized for nine weeks after the incident. When she came home from the hospital, the little girl had no head or trunk control, slept about an hour at a time, and could drink only half an ounce of liquid. A chiropractor, who was also a family friend, applied Cranio-Sacral Therapy. Ginette noticed that the treatment seemed to help. This observation led her to seek more information about CranioSacral Therapy and The Upledger Institute's therapy programs from the Institute's website. Eliane attended her first intensive therapy program in September 1997, three weeks after coming home from the hospital.

"After the first program, Eliane started oral feeding and could drink eight ounces. She started sleeping three and four hours at a time. And, for the first time, I noticed Eliane focus her eyes on someone. It happened when her physical therapist was working on her," Ginette says.

When they returned to Canada, Ginette and her husband Michel, a chiropractor, had Eliane's feeding tube removed. They also decided to slowly decrease the seizure medication prescribed for their daughter because the seizures had stopped. Eliane continued receiving CranioSacral Therapy twice a week, as well as chiropractic and Feldenkrais® sessions. But there was never a doubt that Eliane would return to UI HealthPlex to continue her progress.

"CranioSacral Therapy is something we can focus on and see results," Ginette says.

That's worth a whole field of buttercups.

Community Backs Boy's HealthPlex Visit

July 1998—Kenny's mother, Pat, got a very special gift for Mother's Day this year. Kenny was taking food by mouth for the first time in his young life after a two-week intensive therapy program at the UI HealthPlex clinic. The youngster, who turned six at the end of May, was born with a cranial nerve dysfunction that impaired his breathing, swallowing and vocal abilities.

"It's a dream come true," Pat says. "We've been working for this for nearly six years. Because he missed bottle-feeding and working up to chewing food, we have a lot to work on. But by developing the ability to eat and drink, he hopefully will be able to talk."

Until now, Kenny had been getting his nutrition from a gastric tube. Doctors were stumped by Kenny's condition because all his test results were normal. They recommended physical, occupational and speech therapy, but he hadn't made much progress. Pat read about cranial nerve dysfunction in one of Dr. Upledger's books and thought that CranioSacral Therapy could be helpful. Referrals from other therapists led them to CranioSacral Therapy practitioners near their home in Prospect Park, Pennsylvania.

"Since Kenny began having CranioSacral Therapy about a year

ago, he started learning sign language and showed other improvements," Pat recalls. "His therapists felt he would benefit from the intensive program at The Upledger Institute HealthPlex." But when the family's insurer wouldn't pay for therapy in Florida, their hopes began to turn to disappointment. Pat's brother stepped in and did a thirty-two-mile run as a fundraiser. The run, other events, and donations paid for the therapy program.

"It was a tribute to Kenny to see how many people were willing to give their time and money to help him," Pat says. "If they had never heard of Upledger and CranioSacral Therapy—many of them hadn't—they have now."

With so many people taking an interest, Pat was anxious to return home after the therapy program to share the news about Kenny's progress. He had made gains in all areas—emotional, social, physical, and mental—according to his mother.

Now she hopes that Kenny, through continued therapy, will develop the skills to enjoy all that life has to offer. "I'm striving to give him a piece of birthday cake and treat it like it was his first."

CranioSacral Therapy Is a Family Affair

April 2000—For Osa, a Native American descendant, and her four children, CranioSacral Therapy "has been of enormous physical and spiritual value," she says. Each member of the family has undergone CranioSacral Therapy—for reasons that range from health maintenance, to help with a learning disability, to alleviation of nearly debilitating medical conditions. In each case the improvements have been distinct, if not dramatic.

Osa and her family were first introduced to CranioSacral Therapy in 1994 while on a retreat at a Montana ranch. A friend suggested it for then four-year-old Oge who has Erb's palsy—a paralysis of the upper arm region caused by birth injury. "We tried conventional medicine for years and found that it didn't work," Osa says. "So we decided to try CranioSacral Therapy."

The results were significant following his first treatment. Osa explains, "The pain in his arm was reduced, and he found it loosened his shoulder, which had always been extremely tight and knotted due to the palsy." The session left Oge with a new confidence. "I'm going to ride a horse all by myself when I turn seven," he told Tag, the ranch owner.

Later that same year, Osa brought Oge to The Upledger Institute HealthPlex clinic for a week of intensive therapy with Dr. John Upledger and Dr. Lisa Upledger. "The results were nothing short of incredible," Osa says. Before his treatments, Oge could barely walk without stumbling—also the result of birth trauma, she believes. "After Lisa worked on him," she adds, "not only did he walk well, but he started to run. He plays soccer now!"

Since that time, each member of the family has experienced the benefits of CranioSacral Therapy—perhaps none so profoundly as Osa herself, who has a history of severe spinal problems. As recently as early 1999, she arrived at The Upledger Institute barely able to walk due to acute back spasms and spinal compression following a snowboarding accident. After a week of treatment she walked unassisted onto a plane for her flight home. Osa calls the healing that has taken place within herself and her family "remarkable ... a gift."

Oh, and that promise Oge made to his friend Tag back in 1994? True to his word, Oge returned to that Montana ranch and rode a horse all by himself on his seventh birthday.

Hope, One Step at a Time

November 1999—Imagine a doctor telling you that your child has cerebral palsy. How would you react?

"Trauma, disbelief and anger" are the emotions that overwhelmed Trina Bigham when she learned her seven-month-old son Brennan had cerebral palsy. Robin, who went through a similar experience, added, "The entire family suffered." Her life was changed forever when her daughter Emily was diagnosed with cerebral palsy at two months of age.

Cerebral palsy is notoriously difficult to treat. Although hardly anyone dares to hope for improvement, one never gives up. Yet today, after years of searching, both Robin and Trina state that CranioSacral Therapy has helped their children. And from their perspectives, the benefits have been dramatic.

"You learn early on to stop expecting miracles," Robin says. Her best advice is to be realistic, find what works, and don't close your mind to anything.

Robin started her beloved Emily—who recently turned four years old—with CranioSacral Therapy in November 1998. Part of Emily's cerebral palsy manifested as kyphoscoliosis, a curvature of the spine that impairs stature. Shortly after beginning CranioSacral Therapy, Emily seemed to grow three inches taller.

Trina says that when her son Brennan, now eight, started Cranio-Sacral Therapy, the first benefit she noticed was his new ability to walk with crutches. Prior to that, mobility was not a realistic hope.

Both women are Massachusetts residents and dedicated parents committed to improving their children's health and well-being—preferably through non-invasive methods. And they both recently spent a week at The Upledger Institute HealthPlex Clinical Services to procure intensive therapy for their children.

"Emily had a lot more energy afterward," Robin says. "She was able to walk without her crutches a lot more and for longer distances. She even started running. And she's still getting taller. There are other little things I notice, too, like her nose is more defined. Her facial features are coming out and there are fewer restrictions in the movement and expressiveness of her face."

Trina says that watching Brennan "trying hard to help himself" touches her heart. "I believe CranioSacral Therapy has the potential to help my son be independent. And I believe it will help him connect with his own Inner Physician and help him heal himself."

Progressive, positive results—not miracles—that's what both women are seeking. CranioSacral Therapy has given them that, and they're confident this process of steady, gradual improvement will continue.

They are content to measure their progress—and hope—one step at a time.

Women and War: Post-Traumatic Stress Disorder Crosses All Gender Boundaries

January 2000—Heidi was suffering but she didn't realize it. "Loneliness, depression, isolation, lousy relationships—they were all part of everyday life," she explains. She had lived like that since 1970 when she finished two tours in Vietnam as a combat-hospital nurse. "I was so scarred, I didn't even know it was possible to live without the pain." Her solution: lose herself in long hours of hospital work. She says, "If I kept going and going, I didn't have time to acknowledge the war inside my head."

Then in 1991 at a Veterans Administration hospital, she met a fellow veteran, Jim Shanahan, who described the same nightmares, the same torment, the same horrifying flashbacks. He admitted he'd received nothing but medication to muffle the pain—until he discovered an answer, a way out.

Jim told Heidi they were suffering from post-traumatic stress disorder, or PTSD, and that the answer for him was CranioSacral Therapy—a hands-on approach that had left him feeling better than he had in years. Jim subsequently invited Heidi to join him as a participant in the first two-week PTSD intensive program at The Upledger Institute HealthPlex clinic. But now she faced another fear. CranioSacral Therapy had worked for Jim. But would it work for her?

"The fear of not knowing was even worse than the hell I was living," Heidi says. Yet she knew she wasn't getting help anywhere else. According to Heidi, the Veterans Administration didn't even begin treating women for PTSD and other combat-related ailments until the 1990s.

So Heidi made the commitment. She affirmed her desire—for good health on every level—and headed off to the UI HealthPlex. That's where Heidi discovered just how much denial she had been in. "I had hidden my depression in my work," she says. "But I found out being a workaholic wasn't the problem—it was a symptom. I finally had to admit that PTSD had been making all my choices."

Releasing the hold that it had on her brought a wealth of unexpected dividends: the return of a smile to her face and a curious, forgotten feeling of happiness that would come over her from time to time. Yet it wasn't so much what she was feeling, Heidi says, but that she felt nothing at all. "I had buried my feelings so deep that I felt nothing but flat for years."

Now when emotions arise she deals with them. "CranioSacral Therapy gave me a whole different perspective," she says. "I'm back in control. I make my own decisions and I run my own life."

Heidi tested that newfound sense of security not long ago when she returned to Vietnam with a group of disabled veterans. They biked through the country for two weeks and felt at peace, welcomed by everyone they met. At the end they were ready to return home.

Today Heidi lives in Boulder, Colorado. She has completed advanced studies in CranioSacral Therapy and is now a practitioner. But her biggest change resonates from within. She is a strong, vibrant woman who has transformed her war-torn inner landscape to an oasis of peace.

"I still have night sweats from time to time, and I don't remember my dreams. But now it's okay," Heidi smiles. "After all these years, I'm okay."

Young Dancer Makes Gains, Leaves Past Behind

October 1997—Melissa has not allowed cerebral palsy to limit her life. Her mother, Patricia, has seen the twelve-year-old make tremendous strides during years of physical and occupational therapy—from not being able to walk to getting around on her own with the use of a cane.

When Melissa was dismissed from her physical therapy and occupational therapy programs a few years ago, her parents began to seek other therapies to help her gain more independence. A massage therapist near their home in Tifton, Georgia, told Patricia about CranioSacral Therapy.

"I was skeptical because the concepts of CranioSacral Therapy—that cranial bones move—are contrary to my nursing training," Patricia recalls. "Yet I was hopeful and prayed for a sign that this was the way to help Melissa.

"One week later I talked to one of Melissa's former physical therapists. She had high praise for CranioSacral Therapy. That was the answer we needed."

Before coming for the intensive program at The Upledger Institute HealthPlex, Melissa had a few CranioSacral Therapy sessions in Albany, Georgia. The CranioSacral Therapy practitioner found that Melissa's coronal suture was restricted. Once the coronal suture restriction was reduced, her attention skills improved and Patricia decided to take Melissa off Ritalin®.

Later, when they came to The Upledger Institute HealthPlex for the intensive program, Patricia saw even more changes in her daughter. She stood straighter and walked more smoothly without the cane she used to help her balance. Melissa's upper body seemed stronger; she appeared to vault up on the table when it was time for therapy. Patricia saw emotional changes, too, as her daughter was more comfortable speaking for herself.

Before they left for home, Melissa announced that she wasn't taking her cane because she didn't need it anymore. One more limit had fallen away.

Melissa now enjoys swimming and "Danceability" classes, where she has appeared in recitals for the past two years.

CranioSacral Therapy Brings Quick Relief to Bell's Palsy Patient

April 1997—Imagine waking up one day to find your face paralyzed. Your cheek droops to one side. Your right eye won't close. Your tongue and jaw feel numb.

That's precisely what happened to Tom, but it wasn't just any morning. For him it began last year in Las Vegas—on the first day of a nationwide convention.

"I woke up in my hotel room feeling like I'd slept too hard on my face," Tom recalls. His muscles felt twisted and his neck felt out of alignment. But while his customers that week believed he had had a stroke, a doctor diagnosed it as Bell's Palsy, a sudden and unexplained paralysis that results in distortions of the face.

"He told me they didn't really know what Bell's Palsy was, but he prescribed steroids anyway," Tom says. "They were terrible. They gave me an upset stomach, nervousness, a terrible sense that my whole body was being attacked."

When Tom returned to his home in Palm Beach Gardens, Florida, he immediately went to see Dr. Lisa Upledger, a CranioSacral Therapy practitioner at The Upledger Institute HealthPlex Clinical Services.

"As soon as she touched my face and started putting opposing forces against the muscles, I realized there couldn't be a more perfect treatment for Bell's Palsy," Tom says. "I probably felt fifty percent better after the first visit, not just physically but also psychologically. It was dramatic."

After two weeks' worth of sessions, Tom's condition was almost completely relieved. And he feels like one of the lucky ones.

"Bell's Palsy can last months and months," Tom says, "and some people never lose it. I'll bet ninety-five percent of the people with this condition are never told about CranioSacral Therapy, but it's the first treatment they should look for. Why spend six or seven months with a problem when you can feel better in six or seven hours?"

Our Journey: The Story of My Experience With My Son at The Upledger Institute Intensive Therapy Program

Eileen M. Clark

My son, Sean, my mother and I flew to Palm Beach Gardens, Florida, to attend a one-week intensive therapy program at The Upledger Institute. Sean has been afflicted from birth with birth trauma, a misshapen head and muscular spasticity. The therapy program included CranioSacral Therapy, massage and energy healing. Sean and I were supported by my mother, who lovingly kept us fed at lunch, tended the laundry I forgot about, and ran out for diapers when I forgot those, too.

The following are notes written each day of this amazing journey with my son. As I transcribed the notes, I found myself remembering more. Some passages are taken from my notes, others are comments in present time written as I feel the need to express them. I do not know exactly how this experience affected Sean, although there are many physiological changes that tell a great a story. I'll tell this story from my point of view. However, I believe that Sean spoke through me many times during that week.

General Description of Program and Environment

The therapy room is a large, open space with six tables, the "Pod," and miscellaneous therapy tools. Off to one side is an area with a conference table. Each morning the team of therapists, the six patients and their caregivers meet for "group." The team leader, Ray, lays out any special plans for the day. Each patient or caregiver takes turns sharing their feelings, both physical and emotional. Feedback or questions are shared back and forth. We then join hands in meditation. The therapists then move to the office to prepare for the day while the patients engage in meditation led by Lee, a psychotherapist.

At about 11 A.M. the team comes in and begins work. Each patient has one main therapist for the day. As the day progresses, this therapist might be joined by one or two others. Breaks for water and a brief lunch are fit in between hour-long sessions. Patients receive hands-on treatments on the tables or in individual treatment rooms. They also meet with the psychotherapists. Caregivers either support at the tables, engage in therapy sessions themselves, take ShareCare courses, or spend time supporting each other.

The Pod is a structure built somewhat like a geodesic dome. Inside there is a table. The structure has to be entered through a special opening, but it is not an enclosed room. One can reach through the triangular metal framework. Speakers surround the interior and vibrations can be felt all over the padded table. Music fills the room at all times. Most of the music is "New Age": drumming, African, natural sounds, etc. Lights are either off or kept dim, allowing filtered natural light to enter the mostly glass walls.

Day 1: Monday, July 28, 1997

Evaluations all around the room. Francine begins with Sean. After one hour he sighs "all done" and climbs off the table. Sorry pal, you're not even close to being all done here!

His first session is in the Pod. Drums, heartbeat. Squiggly and wormy at first. Cries out. Something must be happening. Sad to see him uncomfortable, but I know it is doing some good. Now and then he moves his eyes to Francine, then to me—back and forth, checking in with us. Then a knowing look. Calm again. Loving touches to Francine. They seem connected. She begins some mouthwork to loosen frenulum (the membrane under the tongue). Not easy for her to get in. Need the bite stick next time.

4:00 P.M. Intense work on mouth now. Two therapists. He is very quiet. Being held very tightly by both ... almost cradled. Has rough moment, choking, then calm again. Something is happening. Does he understand? Is he ready for this? I think so. I'm staying out of the way. Don't want to distract. I hope he knows I'm near. He is sleeping with this thick stick and a therapist's fingers in his mouth. Really tough stuff. Such a good guy. I love you!

Day 2: Tuesday, July 29, 1997

The Pod! Whoa! Wow! Wow!!! Cathy and Candace work together. I love the Pod. I ask if I can join them. Music plays, with heartbeats, womb sounds, deep vibrations pulsing through the table. I sit next to Sean, touching his stomach. As I listen to the sounds, I begin to talk silently to him. For some reason I tell him that Sue and Darlene (energy healer and old friend) are with us. (Darlene told me later that she felt a "pull" and called to me. We tracked down the day and time. It was exactly at that time!) I feel myself going with him. I see a reddish-orange tube, me at top. Is it Sean down there? I don't actually see him, I just feel as though it is him. I move through the tube to be with him.

Again, silently, "Sean, if I'd only known. If I could have changed it I would've. I'm sorry, Sean." Then I am overcome with tears. They flow and flow. I don't know where all this came from. Cathy tells me to let it go, that I will help him release by doing this. At first I feel such deep sorrow and grief, longing to know where he is and wishing I could have helped him four years ago.

I reach in. "Sean, I'm with you. We are so there. We are so here, Sean!" These words repeat. I think I speak them out loud also. The tears keep flowing and I begin to feel such joy to be with him—with him at the beginning. "We are starting over, from the beginning! We're going to do this, TOGETHER."

During the most intense moments, Cathy touches my back. The position I am in is quite uncomfortable and creates a pain down my back like a tight wire. I realize when it is over, the pain is completely gone!

Such a clean feeling now. He seemed to be asleep throughout. Maybe he was only on another plane or something. I know where he was—I was there too!

When Sean awakens he rises quickly and climbs up to me, clinging like a magnet. Oh, he feels so good to hold.

Candace and Cathy envelop us in their arms, no one speaking, but I can see them communicating and nodding to each other. Sean seems to jump back into the present. We are finished . . . for now. We all climb out of the Pod.

I see each of them holding one end of Sean at the edge of a table. Cathy calls, "Do you have the head?" "Yes," Candace replies. They swoosh him down and off the table. So this is "Rebirthing"?!

(I still get goose bumps when I think of that experience. I describe it as a rewombing. Somehow things are different. While I was never closer to Sean than I was at that time, I think a healthy and necessary separation has occurred. I can allow him to do his work. I don't feel as emotionally hung up with him. Who knows? Maybe today has just been a good day and I'll be a mess again! Dave [my husband] comments that, if I went through all that with Sean, I probably had to leave a bit of baggage behind, as well. I hope so. I hope this new-found peace within me can continue. I know I'll have some crazy days ahead. I only hope for clarity and patience and peace.)

Candace treats Sean for the rest of the day. He is actually falling asleep during sessions. Maybe he'll start to nap better at home.

I have a neuromuscular massage. Ahhhh. Work on trap, head and neck. Love that still point!

Day 3: Wednesday, July 30, 1997

At group we hear about so many wonderful changes for each person. It is tough on me. I don't have any way to know what is happening with him.

I take ShareCare class with Gayle. First a general overview of the craniosacral system, and then learning to feel the rhythm. I have trouble finding it. I'm thinking about Sean. I can't concentrate on the "hands-on." I do find the class interesting, though.

Liza works on Sean. I don't see him until 1 P.M.

I have a good conversation with Ray (the team leader).

Ray reminds me to let Sean do his work. Only he can do it. I can't do it for him. "The bad news is that he is severely restricted. But that is the good news, too!" There is a lot to be done, but there is a lot of potential. HE must decide.

After lunch, I join Liza and Sean. She has me hold him in a tightly compressed position: knees pulled up, arms folded across chest. She works on head and occiput. Lots of sweating and screaming. The frantic red face reminds me of Sean as an infant. The more he screams the more I encourage him on. I don't feel sad for him or guilty for letting him go through this. I know that he is not in physical pain. Part of his outbursts come from frustration at being confined. I sincerely believe that he is experiencing a type of release—pain from the past, anger? It is clear to me that something significant is happening to his body and mind. Whatever it is, I want it to keep going as long as possible. He is so sweaty! Lots of cooking in those membranes! Go, baby, go!

Dr. John Upledger arrives to circulate around the room. I watch him work on Lawrence—six-year-old boy, not sure of diagnosis, ADD maybe. (I befriend his mom. She seems to need some work and support, as well.) Dr. John works; Lawrence protests and cries out. He has exhibited this behavior all week, but his mom is usually out of the room. While holding Sean during Liza's work, I carefully watch Camille (Mom). Liza and I know that hearing Lawrence so unhappy is difficult for her. She begins to cry and moves away from the table. Now is the time to try some energy transfer. We are all put together this week for a reason. Camille needs help. Eventually she pulls herself back in and gets back into the session. Later she tells me that Upledger did a "rebirth" on Lawrence. She says that it was quite a moving experience.

Other patients look as though their bodies are being tortured. Jim has arms and legs being moved in all directions. Rupert appears to be convulsing on the table. Later I ask how they feel. They both say they feel complete peace, trust, no pain at all. Amazing.

Sean's turn. Dr. John at his head, Cathy on Sean's right shoulder area, Liza on left side at feet and back area, Candace on right at sacrum. Dr. John invites me to get on the table with Sean. I choose to sit back and get out of the way.

I have waited six months for this moment. Back when I first read *Your Inner Physician and You,* all I could think of was: If I could only get this guy to hold my child, I know it would work. At the very least I would know that I made every possible attempt to help Sean. Well, here we are—John Upledger only inches away from me and his hands on Sean's head. I must say, though, that after spending three days with the staff, they are extremely effective, competent and gifted in their own rights. I feel a little badly blabbering on about how important it is for me to see Upledger himself. But then again, I had to go to the "Big Kahuna" himself (as Dave says!).

Anyway, Dr. John begins to work on that head. Cathy watches his (Doctor's) face, then closes her eyes, nodding as they work. I know they are communicating with each other. She has told me stories about this. They all work so well together that words are often unnecessary. Dr. John instructs Candace to direct energy from the sacrum up toward the head. Watching his hands is a most incredible experience. He looks as though he is a potter pulling up clay on a wheel. Slowly turning and moving hands upward. He says it feels like popping a cork from a bottle. After awhile he and Cathy almost simultaneously say, "Oh, okay, there it goes!" He then slowly pulls his hands away and hovers them above Sean's head. This man is a healer.

Sean does his usual scramble up to a kneeling position. He lunges toward Upledger. I am so happy. I want so much for him to just hold Sean in his arms for a minute to feel how special this little guy is. (Everyone here at home comes to Sean for hugs when they've had a tough day. He is a little healer himself!) Upledger holds Sean and laughs as Sean dances a little. He hands Sean over to me, thanks me, and walks away. I feel a bit at a loss that I do not have a conversation with him.

The next day at group, I express these feelings. Cathy says that the playful moment with Sean was actually an exception to Dr. John's usual way. Another therapist says that Dr. John sometimes finds verbal expression unnecessary. What needs to be done is done, that's it, move on to the next thing. They experience this in meetings all the time. Okay, I feel better! I feel better to have had him and all these people with my son.

Liza continues into the late afternoon. Joanne joins us. She begins to move more like an energy healer—pulling energy away from his head and tossing it away into the space behind her. Had I not seen Sue Dowling perform this before, I would not understand what is happening. I am so happy that I have witnessed and studied energy work before. I fully understand what they are doing and what they are saying. Liza and Joanne work about the head, mostly the face. Joanne concentrates on his left eye. Does she go there because of the red scar from a bad fall he had taken that spring, or does she just find herself in that place? She feels electricity coming from areas and actually says "ouch!" I love that! I can't stop being utterly fascinated by this stuff!

As they work they give me a lot of narrative. I always appreciate that. I am fascinated by the process and love to hear about the things they are feeling. When you watch CranioSacral Therapy it looks as though they are simply holding the body. Unless you learn about the work you tend to think they are doing nothing.

"I feel the ethmoid dropping. Sphenoid is rocking. Oh yeah, there goes the orbit. Okay, he's pushing me away." (Sean is asleep the entire time.)

The work is done for today. The three of us gently back off. We watch him sleep. We finally have to wake him up. He is definitely ready to get out of there. He cries every time I stop to gather up our gear. Then he becomes a completely happy, vocal, giggly little guy as we stop for dinner and some shopping at a bookstore and T.J. Maxx. In the car I give him the choice of a swim in the ocean or ice cream. He lets out an absolutely clear "CRRRR!" Of course he is a little upset until the goods are produced. It is great to see such affirmative communication. Just to test him out, we walk past the ice cream shoppe. Sure enough, he throws a fit. He knows that is the place!

WHAT A DAY!!! Now that I'm writing it, I can't believe all of what happened. No wonder we are so wiped out!

Day 4: Thursday, July 31, 1997

Ray is Sean's main therapist. He wants to work without me in the room. I make it clear that they should let me know where I should be. He says that he is definitely not shy about telling a caregiver that it is best to leave. At one point he says, "Why don't you go and look at your book?" Okay, got the message!

4:30 P.M. Sitting on opposite side of room from Sean. I'm not happy. I have to go over to that table now!

I go over and Sean immediately climbs up on my shoulder. We

hold close and I just sob. I am sorry for interrupting, but I can't help it. Ray nods and has us both come on the table. Ray has one hand above Sean's head and one hand on my back. I see him toss away some bad energy. Sean will not stay still, but we stay together until the end of the song. I am sorry for breaking in. Ray says that he was about to call me over in a few minutes anyway. Sean has worked hard all day. They tell me that he was cooking (sweating and working) all day but was very quiet. He talks with me a lot about my efforts with Sean, reaffirming and reassuring me that I am doing a lot for him. There will always be more that can be done, but don't burn out.

Lots of important thoughts shared, but no need to recall now for the journal—it's all tucked in my heart and soul. It won't be forgotten.

We say good-bye for the day. As we are packing up, Ray comes to me and shares some wild stories related to energy work. He goes over two of the exercises that I tried while reading a book on the chakra system. I actually feel the energy passing between my hands! It feels like tiny electrical charges passing from the fingers on one hand to those on the other! It never worked before. "If you think it works or think it doesn't, you are probably right." These words come back to me often.

Note: 8/19/97. Since I've been home I've tried a few times to do the energy exercises and nothing has happened. I'm sure it has a lot to do with my focus on so many linear issues. At Upledger my entire focus was toward the spiritual and physical experiences in that room. There truly was an extraordinary amount of energy about the space. I now fully acknowledge the power of being surrounded by people with these abilities. I also found out that I have some of these abilities myself. I just have to focus in order to find them. One of these days when the house is quiet and I'm alone, I'm going to call it up.

Day 5: Friday, August 1, 1997

The last day of this journey.

Waking up I have to write this immediately.

Last night Sean took a long time to settle down. I usually put him to bed and then spend time with my mother in the living room. By the time I am ready for some bedtime reading, he is asleep and I can read in bed next to him. At about 10 P.M. last night, though, I came in and he was still awake. I tried to read and he squirmed and marched happily around the room. I gave up reading and turned out the lights.

As I was dozing off, I suddenly felt the top of his head crash into my forehead. I expected him to move away right after bumping into me. He stayed there, pushing his head into mine. It was so strange. It seemed to be no accidental bump in the dark. Keeping in mind the quote earlier that day about "if you think it is or isn't you are right," I decided to try to remain open-minded and go with this, whatever it was. I thought, okay, Sean, what is it?

With my eyes closed I began to see a circle of light opening. Okay, I don't deny this, keep going. The circle opened and I could clearly see his right ear! Then it closed up. Hmmm, ear. Chloe worked on that ear that morning. I have no idea what that was about. I guess it will dawn on me one day.

Sean and I then parted. He then climbed back over me. I was lying on my left side. He climbed over me near my stomach and headed up toward my face. No big deal. We all enjoy climbing around and snuggling. This time, though, he moved his head around my face as though he were aiming. I say this because he reached the side of my face and planted there the same way he did earlier. He may have fallen asleep. His breathing sounded that way. I started feeling claustrophobic as my face was between his and the pillow. I tried to stay in this position, feeling that he was trying to send some message again. After awhile I couldn't take it anymore and had to move him away. Another weird experience!

Joanne works with Sean in the Pod. They do some mouthwork. "He did some good work" is the general response. No details. Today, though, I can let him go, let them do their thing with him.

Gayle teaches us how to find the craniosacral rhythm in Share-Care class. My mother is the demonstration model for the energy work. She has had shoulder pain for a year or more. Gayle has her show how high she can lift her arm without pain. It looks to be about forty-five degrees. Gayle works on her using a soft touch of her hand, transmitting energy to the area of pain. She tells my mother to completely let go. She relaxes so well that it takes three people to support her. When she lifts her shoulder again it rises to about ninety degrees!

For still point induction Gayle asks for a volunteer. I jump at the chance. I feel like I am falling back inside my head . . . falling and turning. Gayle says, "She's unwinding the dural tube." I hear my mother ask if I feel it. I hear her but have absolutely no desire to talk or move. I am floating and turning. Ahhhh.

Sean is so happy today. Wow! For the first time I do not cry! Well, a tiny bit when Jim and Rupert compliment Camille and me for being "wonderful mothers." We laugh because Camille is also pleased that she hasn't cried until that moment. I hand her some tissues and say that I have gotten into the habit of filling my pockets with them just before group each day. Sean is quiet for the most part during the discussion and then becomes very vocal as we join hands and meditate. While I am embarrassed at his noise during a quiet time, the therapists feel it is remarkable that he is most vocal during that particular moment.

The big Wow! of the day comes when Lee, the psychotherapist, brings Sean into her office for "sand play." This is a form of therapy used with children. In her office stands a cabinet filled with small toys, figurines, ornaments, etc. The children go to the cabinet and take out anything they want. They bring these items to the sand table and play as they wish. The theory is that the children will reveal their soul, fears, hopes, troubles, etc., through the objects selected and the manner in which they play with them. I would be fascinated to see what Kyle or Cody would do.

Lee brings Sean out to the therapy room and invites me into her office to see what Sean has picked. I walk in and look down. I am in shock. There in the sand appears to be a dolphin! My shock surprises her and I share the information given to me by a psychic. The psychic told me that Sean is of the dolphin frequency. (I must do some research and learn more about this.) I still can't believe this happened. My self-protective and skeptical side says, "I must have shared this with someone this week and they told her, and she did this to make me feel good." But the other side of me says, "Not only would this be unethical, but why would they bother?" Lee explains that Sean chose the dolphin and then turned away without taking anything else. He went over to the window and watched the thunderstorm. He seemed very pleased when she opened the window for him. She said that she never watched the rain quite that way before. She wanted us to take the dolphin home. She said that, for her, a dolphin represents peace, resurrection, hope, and intelligence.

Other items that he chose later were: a pink tree, representing spring, hope, and life; a crystal in the shape of a treasure chest. (It was clear but with a gold lock on it. Hmmm); and a figure of a male in green pants and red shirt. Around his waist is a belt and bullets. He has one hand on his hip and the other hand is outstretched and holding a gun. This one throws me off a bit. I ask her what that could be about. She asks me what I think. Maybe fear, protection, fearlessness, power? I will not be surprised one day when it all comes out in the open. I have some confidence that Sean is not a violent person in his soul.

The day ends with a formal re-evaluation by Francine. Sean shows reduction in restrictions throughout. A copy of the report will be sent to us. They recommend that we consider having his frenulum clipped in order to help free up the mouth and the membranes associated with that area. No argument from me! I am happy to have someone suggest it. Two years ago, and again one year ago, we wanted to do it, but oral, motor and speech therapists guarded against it. I tend to agree that he did not have enough muscle tone in his mouth at the time. Now is the time.

A warm and tearful good-bye to everyone. I think we will return.

Note: That night as I was showering with Sean, I noticed the vertebrae in his back had changed. He is a bony guy and the bones in his back always poked out quite a bit. It wasn't a real issue. It just looked odd. Well, those bones were straight and the protrusion GONE!

Saturday, August 2, 1997

The most noticeable developmental change has been in Sean's gait. He once walked with feet spread about shoulder-width apart. His feet are now an inch or two apart and parallel.

Another physical change has been the vertebral shift mentioned earlier.

His head has changed. I'll do some photo comparisons. Others have testified to it. I believe it, but I'm with him so much that it is difficult to see. To me, it seems as though his head curves upward in back. It used to go straight back.

I can't help but feel that Sean is calmer and slower. His sensory system seems more organized. He is more likely to try to communicate in any way he can before crying. He uses his signs and sounds more frequently. When he is ready for a meal or snack he calmly communicates or sits in his chair. He used to cry and head to the snack cabinet, panicking if it was locked.

Dave is astonished by the change in Sean's head. He tells me that he took mental measurements before we went to the clinic. His head has definitely changed shape. When I lifted Sean's shirt and showed Dave the spine, his jaw dropped! I guess this was not my imagination. We watched Sean walk down the hallway and, yes, his feet are closer together than before. Dave and I gave each other a big high-five that night! It was worth every penny and every moment.

Chapter Nine

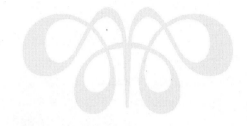

Testimonials

In this concluding section I would like to step aside and let practition-
ers and clients who have been helped by CranioSacral Therapy, Somato-
Emotional Release, and related therapies speak for themselves. First,
Don Ash, a physical therapist trained in CranioSacral Therapy, will tell
us about an important general topic: the healing crisis. Then I want to
present a few of the many letters we have received from clients over the
years at the Institute. Some of them are people I worked with person-
ally. Others are clients of therapists trained at the Institute. Finally I
want to share with you a letter that a client sent, not to me but to her
insurance company as part of her attempt to get it to cover her thera-
peutic costs. I think it may be encouraging and instructive to many
people who face similar struggles.

On the Healing Crisis
by Don Ash, P.T., CST-D

I was reminded by a patient today about the phenomenon of "the healing crisis." It refreshed memories of my own healing crisis and essentially the healing that took place because of it. In my case, I was working
as a physical therapy director of rehab services in a small hospital, but
also as a part-time home-care therapist, columnist for a local news-
paper, school-board member, volunteer fireman, sheep farmer, husband, and father. To say I was unable to recognize that my life was too
hectic is an understatement—so my body tried to help me.

In order for me to see the light, my body gave me a healing crisis. First I came down with gallbladder disease. So I said, "Okay, take it out and I'll stay home a couple of weeks, but then I gotta get back to business." I went back to my schedule and came down with mononucleosis. "Okay," I said, "I'll rest a couple of weeks, but then I gotta get back to work. I've got places to go and people to see."

Then my body became more impatient. I came down with pneumonia and I couldn't breathe. My body was telling me I had to change or go home. No amount of medication or medical intervention in the past twelve months had been able to persuade my body to stop trying to get my attention. By the way, the pneumonia forced me to cancel participation in a continuing education course on fascial release work. If someone had looked at my life as it was at that time, they would have seen a very successful, committed, highly functioning individual who was taking part in his community and prospering. But the fact was that my life was killing me.

I finally realized I had to alter my life. I was doing too much, moving too fast, and not taking time to balance my life with work, rest and play. My wonderful body wouldn't stop until I learned this lesson. It needed the length of time it took to break me down. My recovery from pneumonia also coincided with the next available class of fascial release work in my area. The year was 1987, and it was sponsored by an institute I hadn't heard of before: The Upledger Institute. So began a process of healing that forced me to redirect my life.

I now know that moving from my very data-based, high-stress, institutional setting to having a small CranioSacral practice in an old farmhouse brought me full circle. Had rapid recovery from my physical problems been achieved with medications, I might not have had the time I needed to process the stress factors in my life, nor discover my passion for the work known as CranioSacral Therapy.

A more general lesson I was able to learn as a healing facilitator is that it's okay if some patients don't have immediate positive responses to treatment. They may be in a healing crisis. Their bodies may need the therapist to be unsuccessful in order to allow them more time to process the issues of their life. Pain may be a gift from the body encouraging them to change. If we never knew pain, how would we know pleasure? If we never learned bad, how could we recognize good? If we didn't have night, how could we know the absence of darkness is day? How arrogant we are to think we know what releases need to be released and what emotion needs to be emoted for the greatest good of the patient, and at just what time and place these things are to occur!

Sometimes the very best we can be is present; the best we can do is listen with our hands and facilitate the patient's body to do what it needs to do. It is well to realize that sometimes the best thing we can do for the patient is nothing at all. Wish him a happy life and move on. In other words, being of no help may be exactly what the patient needs at the time.

As we interact in a patient's life, it serves us well to realize that we are simply somewhere along his or her path of life. Whether we are on the path or at the crossroads is the great mystery that can only happen when we observe the present moment. Sometimes it is our role to encourage the body to show the person the beginning or the end of their path. It is the young, expectant mother's healing crisis that causes her cervix to finally give way and the uterus to reach a threshold that begins contractions in an effort to expel the fetus. Sometimes it is the fetus who has a hesitancy to come out of its place of comfort and shelter.

As a physical therapist specializing in CranioSacral Therapy, I occasionally am asked to try CST on an infant that is considered helpless. These young souls all have trouble landing here on earth. I consider them great teachers, considering the fact that most of them are less than six months old and have already confounded the greatest medical centers in the world by their very survival. I held one little man expected to die in the first week of life. He was born with severe anoxia (lack of oxygen to the brain) after a forty-hour home delivery. He required oral suction every twenty minutes. When I held him he was nine weeks old. He came to a still point, arched his neck, and moaned for twenty minutes. His moan was a heartache and sorrow for his circumstances. He moaned like an old woman who had just lost a son in the war. It came from his solar plexus. His lips puckered, his brow furrowed, his fists clenched, and his little body stiffened. He moaned for his circumstance and then for his right to exist. All of us in the room (his mom, other therapists and myself) felt a chill in our spines as he voiced his healing crisis. He is now a year and a half old, moving on all fours. His eyes track. He laughs. He coos. And who's to say he won't live and continue to teach us how precious life is.

Sometimes a healing crisis is the entrance to our exit from life here on earth. As it is related to transition, a healing crisis sometimes occurs to allow the notion of death to descend upon the person. You know when there is no more life left to live. Death (or the transition to another existence) is a wonderful alternative to lingering, suffering and progressive loss of function. When a person is worn down by age or infirmity, fatigued by sleeplessness, and exhausted by struggling for breath, there is a gentle curtain that descends and the person quietly resigns. Struggle stops. Pain and the grimacing face subsides and softens. The mind moves from conflict to acceptance, and visions seem to transcend physical space. Often the person in process sees beyond this physicality and describes the great mystery beyond as bright, warm and pleasant, with friendly, loving faces awaiting.

The healing crisis is the catalyst for an awareness shift in that the stimulation doesn't quit until the patient dies, and then there is calm, peace and transition. And from firsthand-witness experience I can tell you that, after the last breath and after the heart stops, the last physically perceivable movement in the entire body is the cranial rhythm that trails off to a whisper and is gone.

The Chinese express crisis with two symbols, one for danger and one for opportunity. The lesson here is that we are charged as Cranio-Sacral Therapists to stand with patients in the perceived moment of risk and watch for the opportunity to understand and experience this life. Ours is not to know if they are coming or going, only that it is sacred.

David's Talking Very Well, Thank You!
by Phillip Henderson, C.M.T.

In June 1995, three-year-old David Henderson had a stunning break-through at UI HealthPlex's intensive program for learning-disabled children. In his treatment, we used only CranioSacral Therapy and energy cyst release. This is his father's report on the family's experience and David's year of progress.

Saying these words so casually and confidently is the result of a year of great progress, wonderment and appreciation. Before June 1995, my son David could only say one word: "da." Now he verbally expresses his own thoughts, feelings and experiences with comfort and ease.

But let's go back to the beginning. David was born in May of 1992, two months after his mother was involved in a serious auto accident. At birth, David's head was unusually red and asymmetrical. This evolved into a severe right lateral strain with numerous facial restrictions.

Our whole world was turned upside down, the joy and excitement dampened by our fears and anxieties. The dysfunction and struggle during David's first three years was painful and exhausting—so many questions unanswered.

During this time I was studying CranioSacral Therapy and Somato-Emotional Release.

As I learned new skills and techniques, I developed a deep appreciation of the osteopathic care David received as his doctor, Carlisle Holland, D.O., gently and carefully balanced David's head back into symmetry. David would stabilize, but then the right lateral strain with the facial asymmetry would return again and again! David's attitude, behavior and self-esteem all reflected his ongoing trauma and discomfort. His frustration coupled with his inability to manifest verbal expression was heartbreaking.

We exhausted all manner of conventional medical approaches to

David's condition. Brain mapping, pediatric neurology, pediatric neurodevelopment, evaluation, MRIs, speech therapy, etc., yielded lots of analyses with no significant improvement.

Our questions were never truly answered. Raised expectations when we were told that our son David was "gifted and intelligent" gave way to crushed hopes with a diagnosis of "verbal expression dysfunction" and the recommendation to learn sign language. That was the most unacceptable thing of all to us, that David would probably only be able to communicate through sign language.

But as we went through all this as a family, we unknowingly were gaining strength through adversity. When a family member is ill, the whole family can become ill. It's an emotional roller coaster of endless unknown possibilities that wears you down on a daily basis. We were struggling, yet somehow surviving.

I remember a friend asking what the greatest thing would be that could happen to me in my life. I answered with a tear in my eye, "To hear my son say 'Daddy.'" Depression and frustration became more prevalent in our family dynamics. Confidence in finding help was fading quickly.

Regrouping by necessity and yearning for heaven knows what, maybe a miracle, we arrived at UI HealthPlex Clinical Services for the first Learning-Disabled Children Intensive Program. During the next five days, our family experienced love, compassion, deepest fears, then ecstatic joy as David broke through and began saying short sentences! It's important to note that as much as David got out of the clinical experience, my wife Julie, daughter Dana (age 8), and I also had breakthroughs. The experience helped to mend the family dysfunction we were suffering as a result of our ordeal. It was incredible to experience the therapeutic process working for the family as a unit, as well as on each individual.

Children are great mirrors of truth. Observing Dr. John work on David, Dana drew a picture of his hands and wrote the words, "Love passes through." From then on, I've described CranioSacral Therapy as a way of using the hands to allow love to pass through.

After the Learning-Disabled Children Intensive Program, a shift from constant anxiety to looking forward with hope began to take shape for the whole family. David's demeanor changed from one of frustration to enthusiasm as he continued to utter three- and four-word sentences. Dr. John advised: "David has everything he needs to know in the back of his head. Let him be free and love him. Let him teach himself how to talk without limits that might be imposed by continued speech therapy or medical treatment."

Over time, David has continued to improve by leaps and bounds. I was struck recently when, talking with him on the phone, I realized he made himself clear without the advantage of lip reading and body movements!

As time gives perspective, we are all still unwinding and healing. It's a great feeling. Learning to let go of the deep-seated fears and anxieties makes room for love, compassion and harmony.

Meanwhile, David's talking very well, thank you.

Duane M. Tester, Executive Director, Michigan Center for Continuing Education in Osteopathic Medicine

In 1981 I had the occasion to treat Duane M. Tester, director of the Michigan Center for Continuing Education in Osteopathic Medicine, for a head injury he had suffered during a car accident. His head had crashed into the windshield leaving him with a detached retina of the left eye. I used CranioSacral Therapy and SomatoEmotional Release, and also treated him for an energy cyst.

Dear John:

First of all, I want to thank you for developing, conducting, and presenting at the Continuing Medical Education program, "Alternative Manipulative Treatment Approaches," April 11–12, 1981. We had very good comments about the program. Most importantly, I want to thank you for the treatment you gave me on Saturday afternoon. You cannot possibly know the feeling I had when I awoke this Monday morning. It was just as if my eye wasn't even there. I had no sensation of discomfort. It made me feel like a heavy burden or weight was gone from my head and shoulders. The excitement of living and doing returned. The release of "whatever" I have been carrying since my eye accident and, more significantly, since the repair of my detached retina was nothing short of miraculous. I feel so good! And I realize how heavy and depressing the pain and discomfort was by relating to how I now feel. Thank you, friend, for releasing "whatever" and restoring me to my old self.

The reactions I had during your treatment are not easily identified; however, I did experience what seemed to me to be a low-voltage spark on the bridge of my nose and a brief, light tingling in my right hand during cranial manipulation. Other than feeling that I was seeing better out of my right eye immediately upon getting off the table, and having a freer motion in my neck and shoulders, that was about it. As you know, Sunday I was stressed and had a great deal of discomfort while at the Center. I went home at 2 P.M. and just sat back and let it happen. It was quiet and peaceful; a slow and easy evening. I went to bed about 1 A.M. and slept well. I woke up at 8:45 with this great relief of pain and discomfort.

I really looked forward to today, rather than "how much longer will it take?" I wanted to accomplish, to achieve. The force that had engulfed me, focusing upon the discomfort, etc., had disappeared overnight; I had a positive attitude about my existence. I am aware that I can't see out of the left eye, and that it must heal, but now it feels as if there are no restrictions or discomfort in that healing process. WAHOO!

I've rambled on—attempting to give you some insight into my reaction to your treatment. I hope you can gather some meaning out of it all. But know my gratitude for what it has done for me. Thank you.

As ever,
Duane M. Tester
Executive Director

Playing Jazz With the Body:
A CranioSacral Healing Experience

I treated Molly Vass-Lehman after she had suffered a dislocated jaw and damage to her inner ear during a freak accident in a dental chair. I used CranioSacral Therapy, SomatoEmotional Release, and Therapeutic Imagery and Dialogue. Ms. Vass-Lehman writes:

I have to admit that I have never really liked jazz music—that is, until now. It is interesting what roads we are led down to the ground of our own healing, and certainly jazz seemed the most unlikely of routes. There is a dance with life that takes us to unexpected places, and this one brought me to the doorstep of a jazz musician, John Upledger. Most people in the field of alternative medicine know him from his pioneering work in CranioSacral Therapy and his research in bio-mechanics. I came to John after a year of searching for a way to return to normal health. Of course I know that on some level I will never return to normal—where I was before the injury to my jaw and inner ear. We can never go back when we have traveled so far on our inner and outer journey of healing.

When faced with injury or illness, it first seems unbearable that we cannot return to the familiar, the place we have known as the home in our bodies. For me this was the most difficult part—resist-ing the fact that things had changed. I liked my home in my body. I liked the feeling of full function, good energy, and most of all I loved not having to think much about this miraculous thing that worked day in and day out, reliably allowing me to do anything that I wanted to do. All of that changed in a flash after two hours in a dentist's chair when my jaw was dislocated and the force from a simple preventive dental procedure injured my inner ear. Now I have a vertigo disor-der that affects my vision, balance, memory, and almost every activ-ity in my life.

Out of desperation I had tried many things: water fasting, homeopathic treatments, trips to the Mayo clinic, consultation with the top vertigo specialists in the country, and even traveling to Jupiter, Florida, to see a doctor who put me in a machine called a "Space-ball." I hung upside down and was spun around to try to correct the inner-ear problem. After hanging upside down in this machine I remember thinking how it looked similar to the "time machine" in a television program I watched as a child. Now at the age of forty-seven I was wishing that we had technology advanced enough to travel back in time so that I could go back to the hour before the dental appointment and change my decision to walk in the door. But of course this is not possible, and others have experienced far worse fates than mine and have to live with much greater dysfunction.

Here I am, fourteen months later, lying on the table of a physician, healer and jazz musician, getting ready for our work together. Today I feel like a saxophone and on other days like a piano or a trumpet—but always like a musical instrument as he begins one note at a time, feeling his way until the improvisational song of the body begins to emerge. Dr. Upledger is like Pythagoras, the famous mathematician and musician of the Greek period, who made great discoveries because of his ability to find harmony in what seemed like disharmony.

John Upledger is a genius of the body because he, like all great artists, merges with his instrument, always asking to be led to the next note, never assuming the composition is already written. Artists are geniuses, not only because of their knowledge but also because of their ability to become completely absorbed in the moment of their craft without distraction. It reminds me of the ancient Chinese story of the wood carver who, even under the threat of death, was able to allow all of his physical, intellectual and spiritual energy to come into a one-pointed flow that created the most magnificent bell stand in the land. This kind of artistic genius cannot be imitated. We must each find our own inner wellspring of creation and allow this to burst forth from its place of spontaneity and love.

I am constantly amazed. How does he know today that there is a pain in my second cervical area and left sternum region, when there is a whole body of possibility? Where does this knowledge come from? Is it psychic, a photographic memory of the anatomy of the body, or the years of experience with thousands of individuals? I suspect that it is combinations of all of these and, of course, the mystery of healing itself.

I used to think that I had some idea of what was required for healing, or at least for the prevention of illness, until several of my healthiest friends died at an early age. They had excellent diets, exercised daily, meditated and did all of the things that I thought would help in the prevention of illness. Of course I still believe that healthy lifestyle choices are important because they help us to have a greater vitality with which to enjoy each day of life we are given. But healing is much more mysterious than we can fully understand. And suffice it to say, it seems to do with faith in something we cannot fully know or express.

When we find illness at our doorstep we are catapulted into a new territory without familiar markers. It can be a desert experience. Faith is the element that carries us to the other side, even when we do not know our way. If we are fortunate there may come a time in the process when we can catch a glimpse of the possibility that this illness is a blessing in the larger context of our lives and evolution.

I should say honestly that this is just an "inkling" at this point in my own experience. Many days I just want to be able to function normally. But inklings are powerful and work in ways we cannot fully understand until the miracle of healing emerges. All I know for now is that I have a growing appreciation for jazz; I believe dolphin energy can heal us, as well as the spirit in back of all life; and I am grateful for ending up at the doorstep of John Upledger. I believe that healing is art, science and spirit, and I know too little to try to figure out how much of each of these is at work in the process. It is enough to try to honor the presence of a healing energy. Those who go deep into this mystery often find the blessing.

I am not ready to write a thank-you note to the dentist, but I will know healing has occurred on all levels when I feel an impulse to do so! But I am ready to write a thank-you note to you, John, and to wish you the happiest of birthdays.

Happy Birthday, John

In gratitude, Molly Vass-Lehman

February 10, 2000

Eleanor Mauder

I worked on Eleanor Mauder only one time, at a demonstration of CranioSacral Therapy and SomatoEmotional Release at a class in San Diego. At that time her chief complaints were rib cage, low back and pelvic pain; frequent attacks of dizziness; chronic fatigue; episodes of choking sensations; and urinary incontinence.

Dear Dr. Upledger,

It's been a year now since I returned from seeing you in San Diego. That experience really improved my energy level. The effects were immediate!

That very evening after flying back to San Francisco, I was able to enjoy a visit with my brother and his family until midnight. The following morning I was able to accomplish another of my goals: to go to the ocean and stand in the waves. What a thrill to feel them crashing on my body. The following morning we took the nine-hour drive back to Oregon. The energy was still there.

Things have just continued to improve since then. I'm now totally continent, can do eight push-ups (men's style), garden, bake, and enjoy life to the full. I walk to and from church (about one-third of a mile round-trip) each Sunday and then even have energy to walk my two dogs. The dizziness I used to experience as I turned over in bed is also gone, and the choking experiences are less often and less severe. In fact, I had the first episode in almost three months on Sunday, July 24, as I was walking to church, but I was able to get hold of myself and continue the walk.

My life is back to "regular" living. I rise at 5:30 A.M., pray with my husband till 6:25, and then begin my daily triathlon: riding my bike to the pool, swimming, and then walking my dogs. This is followed by breakfast, quiet time, a visit with my parents, or a trip to the grocery store. I no longer use anything but the grocery cart and can even tolerate waiting in the check-out line.

Lunch is followed by quiet time and then sewing, reading, toy repair, or whatever seems enjoyable at the time.

Friday and Saturday mornings are special. We go garage saling. I get in and out of the van six or ten times, walking to and from the sales. CranioSacral Therapy has helped me stretch my legs to the fullest.

My rib cage is now almost pain-free and I can do fun things and enjoy them!

My husband does CranioSacral Therapy with me daily, so I am most fortunate. I am living proof of the value of this therapy and thank you for the part you have played in my journey.

Sincerely,

Eleanor Mauder

Pamela D. Markert

Dear Doctor Upledger:

I am writing to thank you for all your pioneering work with Cranio-Sacral Therapy. It has made a profound difference in my life both personally and professionally as a physical therapist.

Back in the early '90s my husband and I wanted to start a family. Although I had undergone surgery when I was twelve years old for removal of a paraovarian cyst and one fallopian tube, my doctor did not feel I would have trouble conceiving. After a couple of years of trying, and some medical testing that was negative, I decided to try cranial work. During a pelvic diaphragm release, a restriction along the incisional area was discovered and released. Following that treatment my menstrual cramps became minimal and I no longer needed prescription medication for the pain. We conceived the following month without further intervention of any kind.

During my pregnancy I was plagued by "morning" sickness that lasted twenty-four hours a day. Fortunately for me I was attending a CranioSacral course at the time and received a couple of treatments. My morning sickness disappeared immediately. Following the course it returned somewhat, unfortunately, but I suspect it may have completely abated and not returned had I been able to have a bit more work done. It still amazes me how good I felt after the treatment, when before I felt so awful. I am grateful that the morning sickness never returned to the level at which it had been prior to treatment.

As my pregnancy advanced, I began to develop a constant right-sided headache, as well as tight lumbosacral pain with right-sided sciatica. Although I was working full-time as a physical therapist, it was getting more and more difficult. This time I came down to the Institute to receive three treatments in your clinic. By the end of those sessions I was a new woman! I am pleased to report that the headache, lumbosacral pain and sciatica vanished, never to return. On top of that I could feel the uterus being de-rotated, and it felt as if it was returned to its proper position. The pubic synthesis was opened to allow an easy delivery, which worked. At forty-two-weeks' gestation, I was able to vaginally deliver a nine-pound, five-ounce baby without the use of suction, forceps, etc. I am absolutely convinced this could not have happened without the CranioSacral Therapy.

This past year I was blessed with my second pregnancy, this one occurring the first time we tried to conceive. I was able to carry twins to a forty-week gestation, and both were born a good size and healthy.

I did notice that my son's eye did not track and follow his other eye as he began to grow and develop. At one month I did a cranial evaluation on him and discovered a large right temporal lesion affecting surrounding structures, including his eye and cranial nerves. With a bit of treatment the area released and, within a short period of time, I watched the eye correct. Both eyes are now working in perfect unison. I suspect that, had this problem not been corrected in the early stages of life, it would have led to a much larger problem down the road that may have required surgery.

These are just a few of the benefits my family and I have derived from CranioSacral Therapy. The list would go on and on if I were to list them all. With healthcare reform being such a paramount issue, I truly feel CranioSacral Therapy can aid in the revolutionizing of our healthcare system.

I hope that, as insurance companies work to cut costs and curtail excessive spending, CranioSacral Therapy is seriously considered as a low-cost treatment for women during obstetrics. It certainly allowed this time in my life to be far more comfortable and enjoyable, and reduced the amount of traditional medical intervention needed, thus cutting costs.

My sincere thanks,

Pamela D. Markert, P.T.

Reid Mendenhall

Dear John,

I wanted to write and reflect something of my life that I believe to be directly associated with my experience at the Institute during the two-week Vietnam Veterans Intensive Program of October 1991. To say that my life has been forever changed does not quite put into words what I have experienced since the program ended. There has been an ongoing change that is profound in nature. The benefit from those changes has been for me a wonder, and my thanks to you and your staff cannot sufficiently be put into words.

I can be a little more specific in saying that a depression that had plagued me for some thirty-odd years was severely jolted. The period of depression that would usually start mid-November every year and continue through December failed to appear until February of 2000. That is where it also ended. To date—February 20, 2001—the depression has not resurfaced. I am feeling more like a human being than I can remember. I have joy in my heart and am smiling. I have started back with my artwork, which I hadn't touched in over six years.

To say these are subtle changes, I cannot. I can only say that the quality of my life has steadily improved in subtle time. One man's life has been affected and continues to be affected by the foresight, love and humanity of many.

Sincerely,

From the heart,

Reid Mendenhall

Claims Review

May 21, 1999

Dear Claims Review Committee:

Enclosed please find copies of my itemized medical bills ($6,500) and treatment summary from The Upledger Institute's two-week intensive program in Palm Beach Gardens, Florida. I feel that in order to justify reimbursement of these expenses, I need to describe the last eleven years of my medical experiences.

Eleven years ago, on September 12, 1988, I underwent a vaginal hysterectomy in Wichita, Kansas. Prior to the surgery my surgeon said that I would probably be back to teaching high school within four weeks. However, instead of returning to work mid-October, I missed most of that school year. After my surgery I developed symptoms that included: neck and back pain (specific vertebrae very sore to the touch); overall muscle soreness and weakness; migraine headaches; fatigue, irritable bowel; frequent low-grade fevers and infections; and I had laryngitis for six weeks. On January 21, 1989, the same surgeon performed a corrective laparoscopic procedure to reduce my lower abdominal pain. I was never able to obtain a viable explanation from either the surgeon or my primary doctor for my ongoing symptoms that followed the original surgery.

In 1990 we moved back to Madison, Wisconsin, to be near our family and friends. In addition to the previous symptoms, I now experienced frequent sinus infections, greater muscle soreness and weakness during colder weather, and increased fatigue.

In 1992, three years after my surgery, Dr. Dan Malone, University of Wisconsin-Rheumatology, diagnosed me with fibromyalgia syndrome. For the next four years, with the dedicated support of Dr. Malone, I tried several medical treatments, including various medications, injections, a walking program and changes in diet. Although these traditional treatments helped me manage my symptoms, my overall strength and physical endurance continued to decline.

The fall of 1996 was the last semester that I taught college-level evening marketing courses as an adjunct instructor. I found it very difficult to focus and remember detailed information as the day progressed. Additional symptoms developed, including: acute sensitivity to sunlight and indoor lighting; acute sensitivity to loud noises and changes in sound levels; frequent nausea from normal home and work-environment smells; frequent red, raised rash on my neck, chest and abdomen; and an altered sense of smell and taste, i.e., most foods tasted the same to me. I felt exhausted most of the time.

In February 1977, under the care of Dr. Malone, I went on a six-month medical leave of absence from my full-time position. In March 1997, Dr. John Doyle, University of Wisconsin-Dentistry, diagnosed me with temporomandibular joint syndrome and I was fitted for a jaw splint. The inside of my mouth was continuously dry and became very sore with ridgelike scars.

During the remaining four months of my leave of absence, I participated three to four times a week in warm-water P.T. and land P.T. for muscle strengthening and pain reduction through the UW-Spine Center. In August 1997, Dr. James Leonard, UW-Spine Center, evaluated me. My treatment plan continued with warm-water and land P.T. exercises, psychotherapy and medications. I returned to work mid-August on a part-time basis at fifteen hours per week and gradually increased my hours to twenty-five per week.

Then on February 10, 1998, I was rear-ended by an uninsured motorist. I was taken by ambulance to UW-Emergency for x-rays and evaluation and was instructed to follow-up with my primary doctor. Two days later, Dr. Lorna Belsky, UW-Women's Clinic, examined me. She wrote a referral for me to see Dr. Leonard at the UW-Spine Center for further evaluation and treatment recommendations. I had suffered left hip and whiplash injuries plus a marked increase in migraine headaches (from three to four per month to two to three per week).

These car-accident injuries exacerbated all my previous symptoms. My overall pain increased both in intensity and frequency. In addition, my sleep disturbance pattern worsened and, thus, so did the dark circles under my eyes. New treatments were added to my regimen, including CranioSacral Therapy and iontophoresis. Land P.T. increased to two or three per week. My intake of Imitrex was increased to two or three tablets per week in addition to naproxen.

In the summer of 1998, Dr. Malone, UW-Rheumatology, referred me to Dr. Daniel Haffex at the Chicago Institute for Neurological Research. I endured many diagnostic tests including MRIs, CT scans, x-rays, and a myelogram. In fact, the result of this intensive testing in August 1998 was a recommendation for back surgery, which included removal of bone from five vertebrae in an attempt to reduce my back and neck pain. The estimated cost of this surgery was $41,000. Several months of intensive follow-up rehabilitation were usually required before the patient returned to work.

I was determined to find an answer to my health problems other than back surgery. Fortunately, in the fall of 1998, one of my P.T.s loaned me a book, *Your Inner Physician and You* by Dr. John Upledger, which addressed chronic-pain treatments such as CranioSacral Therapy, SomatoEmotional Release, Visceral Manipulation, neuromuscular re-education, myofascial mobilization and psychotherapy.

After reading the book I contacted The Upledger Institute HealthPlex Clinical Services. I was informed that in order to attend their two-week intensive program, I had to first be evaluated by an Upledger Institute-trained practitioner. In the Madison area my contact for this evaluation was Dr. Ray Purdy. I was treated by Dr. Purdy three or four times per month from October 1998 to March 1999. After a few visits to Dr. Purdy, I ceased all other P.T. and O.T. treatments. His treatments resulted in more pain relief than all other medical services and medications I had tried. These treatments definitely laid the groundwork for the positive changes I would experience at UI HealthPlex.

Filled with hope, my husband and I traveled to Florida for the two-week intensive program, March 8, 1999. I spent approximately seven hours a day on a treatment table at the clinic. (There are only six patients at each two-week intensive program.)

A team of healthcare professionals provided a range of appropriate treatments based on what I felt I needed. The Upledger environment felt safe and nurturing, ideal for my healing process to take place. My husband attended ShareCare® educational workshops, which are designed to inform family members about the two-week intensive program. He enjoyed being part of my daily treatment in a very supportive role.

On the third day of my two-week intensive program at UI Health-Plex, I experienced my first major breakthrough. I finally found out the "TRUTH" about what actually happened to me eleven years earlier during the vaginal hysterectomy. While lying on a treatment table, encouraged by Dr. John Upledger and clinic staff, I was able to verbalize many details of my surgery. It became obvious from these details that I was under-anesthetized during my surgery. In fact, I experienced excruciating pain and a horrific fear of dying. In addition, I experienced intense anger toward the surgeon, anesthesiologist and other operating room staff that they were allowing this to happen to me. Although I was aware of the surgery taking place, I was not able to move or scream due to the anesthesia, restraints, and tube down my throat. I felt trapped while they removed my uterus. I vividly recalled the pain of the sharp surgical knife cutting into me.

I will never forget that Wednesday afternoon experience at UI HealthPlex, specifically my screams of sheer terror as I relived my surgery. Neither will my husband. The realization of what really happened to me was very empowering. This pain had been trapped inside me for eleven years. This pain is now on the outside of me as a past event. The blend of traditional and non-traditional treatments at UI HealthPlex helped me finally make sense of all my ongoing symptoms. The two-week intensive program was definitely a mind-body connecting experience for me!

My second major breakthrough occurred during the last week of this program. Dr. John Upledger and several staff members assisted in a "multiple-hands" adjustment from my pelvic floor up to my head in an attempt to release the pressure in my spine.

The result of their effort is that my spine no longer hurts when touched nor does it radiate pain. I am now my normal height, which is one and a half inches taller than when I arrived at the clinic. Also, my walking gait is now normal.

Even though my spinal pain is gone, I am dealing with residual muscle soreness and weakness, chronic fatigue, left hip flexion-related pain, and memory-triggered emotions, all of which are decreasing every week due to my ongoing recovery efforts. Dr. Leonard, UW-Spine Center, evaluated me one month after I attended The Upledger Institute HealthPlex clinic. We discussed my thoughts on what I needed to do to continue to heal. With Dr. Leonard's dedicated support, my current treatment plan includes:

• Bi-monthly myofascial pain release treatments through Dr. Ray Purdy;

• Bi-monthly neuromuscular therapy through Katie Camp and Associates;

• Weekly warm-water P.T. through Lori Thein-Brody, UW-Spine Center;

• An independent daily walking program;

• Bi-monthly land P.T. through Laurie Sanford, UW-Spine Center;

• Follow-up visits with Dr. James Leonard, UW-Spine Center;

• Psychotherapy sessions, as needed, with Dr. Paul Thoresen;

• Follow-up visits with Dr. James Leonard, UW-Spine Center;

• Yearly physical exam with Dr. Lorna Belsky, UW-Women's Health Center; and

• Follow-up visits with Dr. John Doyle, dentist, for TMJ treatments.

I am immersed in my treatment plan and am highly motivated to regain my pre-surgery strength and lifestyle. My husband Jim, daughter Jennifer, and I are all delighted with my progress.

Since I left UI HealthPlex two months ago, I am continuing to improve and adjust to all the changes in my body and mind. These changes include:

- I now sweat when I walk. I am able to walk briskly for thirty to thirty-five minutes, covering about one and a half miles.
- I have lost twenty-three of the seventy-eight pounds I had gained.
- I now have noticeably more saliva in my mouth and dry mouth symptoms are decreasing.
- My TMJ symptoms have greatly decreased.
- The moisture in my eyes continues to increase and I look forward to wearing contact lenses soon.
- The hair along my facial hairline is growing in noticeably thicker.
- I have a slight blush to my face, which is normal for me.
- I generally feel warm and relaxed.
- My short-term memory and ability to focus have greatly improved.
- I smile and laugh more frequently.
- The only medication I am taking is Imitrex® for infrequent migraine headaches.
- I am filled with joy and optimism. Every day I am closer to "wellness."
- As of May 3, 1999, I have increased my work hours to thirty per week.

During the eleven years prior to attending The Upledger Institute HealthPlex clinic, I was never able to find out what actually happened to me. I am very thankful that, through my experience at the clinic, I now know that the symptoms I presented—indicative of fibromyalgia syndrome and post-traumatic stress syndrome—were in fact caused by my September 12, 1988, surgery.

The treatments I received at the UI HealthPlex clinic during the two-week intensive program were both reasonable in cost and performed out of medical necessity. As documented in this letter, I had diligently tried all the recommended "traditional treatments" without regaining pre-surgery health. Throughout these eleven years I continued to decline in both physical strength and endurance. I also continued to develop additional symptoms. These treatments were most beneficial to me, as evidenced by the absence of spinal pain and measurable reduction in all my other symptoms.

I sincerely hope that this account of my medical experiences proves to be insightful as you review my request. If you have any questions, please contact me.

Sincerely,

Jill L. Mason

Afterword

If you have read the descriptions of the path I have followed and all of the signposts that have guided me along the way, you are to be congratulated. I have no illusion that all of the things I have said in this book will be acceptable to you. I offer my experiences and observations to you, and you can accept those that you find palatable and reject those that are distasteful to you for one reason or another. At this point I can only say that everything I have written is true and has been described to the best of my ability. These happenings and experiences have opened my mind significantly. I have gone from being a hard-line scientist who required proof, to believing that what I see or experience is true, even though I may not know how it happens. I have become a clinical-outcome person who would rather observe and accept what I see than reject an observation, experience or practice because it has not yet been scientifically proven. If it is very low-risk or totally risk-free, and it seems reasonable, I'll try it. After all, if we can't use something until we understand it, then we shouldn't be using gravity.

I hope that your mind is open enough to think freely about the phenomena that have been described in this book.

Index

About the Author

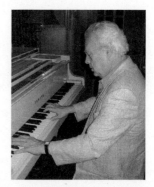

John E. Upledger, D.O., O.M.M.

Dr. John E. Upledger is founder of The Upledger Institute, Inc.® Dedicated to the natural enhancement of health, the Institute is recognized worldwide for its groundbreaking continuing education programs, clinical research and therapeutic services.

Throughout his career as an osteopathic physician and surgeon, Dr. Upledger has been recognized as an innovator and leading proponent in the investigation of new therapies. His development of CranioSacral Therapy in particular has earned him an international reputation.

His work has been featured on *Good Morning America*, *ESPN*, *Oprah* and *CNN*, and in publications such as *USA TODAY* and *TIME* magazine, where he was featured in "TIME 100: The Next Wave," a "look into the future to discover tomorrow's most influential individuals."

Dr. Upledger is a Certified Specialist of Osteopathic Manipulative Medicine, an Academic Fellow of the British Society of Osteopathy, and a Doctor of Science. He has served on the Alternative Medicine Program Advisory Council for the Office of Alternative Medicine at the National Institutes of Health. And in 2000, Dr. Upledger testified before a U.S. Government Reform Committee meeting on the potential effects of CranioSacral Therapy on autism.

Contact Information

For information on healthcare continuing education workshops for professionals and educational materials (modalities include Cranio-Sacral Therapy, SomatoEmotional Release®, Mechanical Link, Visceral Manipulation, Lymph Drainage TherapySM, Therapeutic Imagery and Dialogue, and related techniques):

The Upledger Institute, Inc.®
11211 Prosperity Farms Road D-325
Palm Beach Gardens, Florida 33410-3487

Phone: 1-800-233-5880 or 561-622-4334
Fax: 561-622-4771

Website: www.upledger.com
E-mail: upledger@upledger.com